International Ophthalmology Clinics

International Ophthalmology Clinics (ISSN 0020-8167) (ISBN 0-316-49859-9). Published quarterly by Little, Brown and Company, 34 Beacon Street, Boston, Massachusetts 02108-1493. Send address changes and subscription orders to Little, Brown and Company, Subscription Department, PO Box 2033, Langhorne, PA 19047-9480; (800) 628-4221. Subscription rates per year: personal subscription, U.S. and possessions, $81; foreign (includes Mexico), $105; Canada, $92; institutional, U.S., $99; foreign, $129; Canada, $109. Special rates for students, interns and residents per year: U.S., $55; foreign, $75; Canada, $65. Single copies: $30 for subscribers, $38 for nonsubscribers. In Japan please contact our exclusive agent: Medsi, 1-2-13 Yushima, Bunkyo-ku, Tokyo 113, Japan. Subscription rates per year in Japan: individual, ¥22,200; institutional, ¥26,200 (air cargo service only). Second-class postage paid at Boston, Massachusetts, and at additional mailing offices.

Postmaster: Send address changes to International Ophthalmology Clinics, PO Box 2033, Langhorne, PA 19047-9480.

International Ophthalmology Clinics is indexed in Index Medicus, Current Contents/Clinical Practice, Excerpta Medica, and Current Awareness in Biological Sciences.

International Ophthalmology Clinics

Volume 31
Number 4
Fall 1991

Neuro-ophthalmology

EDITED BY

Lanning B. Kline, M.D.

University of Alabama School of Medicine, Birmingham, Alabama

Little, Brown and Company
BOSTON

Editors

Gilbert Smolin, M.D.

F.I. Proctor Foundation, San Francisco
Department of Ophthalmology,
University of California, San Francisco
Medical Center

Mitchell H. Friedlaender, M.D.

Division of Ophthalmology,
Scripps Clinic and Research Foundation,
La Jolla, California

Editorial Office

931 West San Bruno Avenue
San Bruno, CA 94066

Publisher

Little, Brown and Company, Boston, Massachusetts

Publishing Staff

Publisher
Lynne Herndon

Executive Editor
Christine F. Lamb

Managing Editor
Sherri Frank

Sales and Marketing Manager
Anne Orens

Production Manager
Fredda Purgalin

Editorial Board

Contents

Contributing Authors

Lanning B. Kline, M.D., EDITOR
University of Alabama
School of Medicine
Birmingham, AL
Address correspondence to:
1600 7th Avenue South
Suite 555
Birmingham, AL 35233

J. Donald M. Gass, M.D.
Bascom Palmer Eye Institute
P.O. Box 016880
Miami, FL 33101

Saunders L. Hupp, M.D.
University of South Alabama
P.O. Box 81327
Mobile, AL 36689

John S. Kennerdell, M.D.
Allegheny Ophthalmic and Orbital Center
320 East North Avenue
Pittsburgh, PA 15212

Simmons Lessell, M.D.
Department of Ophthalmology
Harvard Medical School
Massachusetts Eye and Ear Infirmary
243 Charles Street
Boston, MA 02114

John A. McCrary III, M.D.
Cullen Eye Institute, C-207
6501 Fannin Street
Houston, TX 77030

Neil R. Miller, M.D., F.A.C.S.
The Johns Hopkins Hospital
Maumenee B-109
Baltimore, MD 21205

Richard P. Mills, M.D.
Department of Ophthalmology, RJ-10
University of Washington
Seattle, WA 98195

Marian Rubenfeld, M.D., Ph.D.
Veterans Administration Hospital *and*
University of Minnesota
Minneapolis, MN
Address correspondence to:
University of Minnesota Hospital
Box 493
516 Delaware Street S.E.
Minneapolis, MN 55455

Robert C. Sergott, M.D.
Wills Eye Hospital
Neuro-ophthalmology Service
Ninth and Walnut Streets
Philadelphia, PA 19107

J. Lawton Smith, M.D.
Bascom Palmer Eye Institute
P.O. Box 016880
Miami, FL 33101

Jonathan D. Trobe, M.D.
W. K. Kellogg Eye Center
University of Michigan
1000 Wall Street
Ann Arbor, MI 48105

Nicholas J. Volpe, M.D.
Department of Ophthalmology
Harvard Medical School
Massachusetts Eye and Ear Infirmary
243 Charles Street
Boston, MA 02114

Jonathan D. Wirtschafter, M.D., F.A.C.S.
University of Minnesota Hospital
Box 493
516 Delaware Street S.E.
Minneapolis, MN 55455

Preface

The purpose of this issue of *International Ophthalmology Clinics* is to review many of the important developments and issues affecting neuro-ophthalmology during the last decade of the twentieth century. Because changes are occurring rapidly this is a large order, and I am indebted to all the contributors for this excellent material. Their chapters demonstrate how neuro-ophthalmology continues to expand in scope, dealing with a variety of advances including magnetic resonance imaging, botulinum toxin, and optic nerve sheath decompression.

I would like to thank William F. Hoyt, M.D., for his encouragement and guidance in preparing this issue. He continues to teach, inspire, and challenge neuro-ophthalmologists throughout the world.

Neuro-ophthalmology has not been featured in this journal since 1986. I hope this issue succeeds in updating the readers on the current state of the art of our subspecialty.

Lanning B. Kline

The Future of Neuro-ophthalmology

Neil R. Miller, M.D., F.A.C.S.

Neuro-ophthalmology has traditionally been a specialty characterized by observation and clinical diagnosis. When F. Walsh first conceived of such a specialty, he envisioned it as a clinical link among the apparently disparate areas of internal medicine, neurology, neurosurgery, radiology, and ophthalmology. The neuro-ophthalmologist was someone who crossed over into these specialties to the extent that he or she could find the common denominator among a series of apparently unrelated clinical symptoms and signs that included disturbances of visual sensory function, ocular motor function, or both. Walsh, along with D. Cogan and R. Lindenberg, also emphasized clinicopathological correlation as the means to understanding most diseases. Subsequent technological advances have revolutionized our ability to diagnose a host of disorders to the extent that many physicians have predicted that neuro-ophthalmologists as diagnosticians will eventually disappear, replaced by neuroimaging studies and other computer-aided diagnostic tests. I beg to differ. Indeed, the future of neuro-ophthalmology has never looked so promising. In the next decade, I believe that neuro-ophthalmologists will continue to have a major role in the clinical diagnosis of various neurological disorders that affect visual function, and will also continue their roles as teachers, prognosticators, researchers, and, perhaps most important of all, as renderers of therapy.

Diagnostic Neuro-ophthalmology

There is no doubt that the development of computed tomographic (CT) scanning and magnetic resonance imaging (MRI) has dramatically altered the way neuro-ophthalmologists practice medicine. First, the risk/benefit ratio inherent in performing diagnostic neuroimaging studies has been changed. Before CT and MRI, skull radiographs and polytomograms were the only imaging studies that were reasonably safe and simple to perform. Neuro-ophthalmologists who suspected an intracranial lesion in the absence of an abnormal skull radiograph or a set of polytomograms was committing patients to a cerebral arteriogram, pneumoencephalogram, or both. For patients with pupil-sparing oculomotor nerve paresis, a decision had to be made whether it was worth the risk of a cerebral arteriogram to detect an intracranial aneurysm. The relative safety of CT and MRI, even when enhancing agents are used, has resulted in the liberal use of these techniques, even when the likelihood of a treatable intracranial lesion is extremely low. Although this approach may significantly increase the cost of medical care and may result in the fortuitous detection of asymptomatic lesions, resulting in the need to determine how to treat such lesions, who is to say at what level of probability it is inappropriate to perform a safe study? If a patient has a 1 in 100,000 chance of having a treatable lesion, and the study used to detect it has no risk, is it not appropriate to perform the study? In addition, the tendency of the public to believe that any unexpected or bad result is deserving of financial compensation has forced almost all diagnosticians to practice what has been called "defensive medicine." The combination of safe, simple imaging studies and an increasingly litigious society virtually guarantees widespread use of such studies in the future.

Future improvements in CT scanning will include the increasing use of both two-dimensional and three-dimensional imaging, both for diagnosis and in the operating room to localize lesions. Improvements in MRI will include thinner sections, faster scanning time, improved paramagnetic contrast agents, and, like CT, increasing use of three-dimensional imaging for both diagnosis and localization. In addition, MR angiography, which permits a reasonable view of both intracranial and extracranial arteries and veins without the need for intravenous or intraarterial injections of contrast material, should improve with respect to both contrast and clarity.

Improvements in our ability to test visual sensory function have been slow and less impressive than most of us had hoped. Contrast sensitivity testing, using a variety of techniques, seems to provide some degree of increased sensitivity for visual sensory function; however, the amount of information gained compared with that obtained from simple testing of visual acuity is unimpressive.

Automated, static perimetry has some very definite advantages over nonautomated, kinetic perimetry. Increased sensitivity and reproducibility are two of the most important advantages. Perimetry still suffers, however, from requiring too much time. The future will provide us with fast, equally sensitive means of testing the visual field.

Color vision remains an important method of testing visual sensory function. Attempts at combining testing of color perception and visual field have not been universally accepted, but such psychophysical tests will become more streamlined and standardized in the future.

Despite the myriad of tests that are and will continue to be available for testing of visual sensory function, our methods of testing vision are woefully inadequate. We must improve the sensitivity of our testing in the future. In addition, simply having such tests available in no way insures the tests will be performed or will be performed correctly. J. L. Smith has emphasized that most mistakes in diagnosis of neuro-ophthalmological problems (and, indeed, of most diseases) occur from the "sins of omission" and the "sins of commission." Physicians either don't perform the appropriate studies, or the studies are performed or interpreted incorrectly. As long as this happens, the future of neuro-ophthalmologists as diagnosticians seems assured.

■ Teaching Neuro-ophthalmology

It is fascinating how many neuro-ophthalmologists have been honored with teaching awards. It would seem that those of us who have chosen neuro-ophthalmology as a specialty have also embraced teaching as one of our goals. We teach at all levels: to patients, students, residents, fellows, practitioners, and peers. Our responsibility to teach will increase in the future as it becomes increasingly important to provide patients and physicians with the latest information in areas that cross subspecialty lines.

The educational responsibilities of neuro-ophthalmologists are not now and will not be limited in the future to neuro-ophthalmology. Many of us are already involved in or in charge of resident selection and resident education committees. With increasing emphasis on the importance of financial remuneration in academic institutions, neuro-ophthalmologists must remind those who have forgotten of the importance of teaching in this environment, even if it is not financially rewarding. We can spread more knowledge and ultimately help more patients by teaching than by examining and treating individual patients.

■ Prognostic Neuro-ophthalmology

Because of the improvement in diagnostic techniques, many patients referred to neuro-ophthalmologists have already had a diagnosis made. They are referred for a complete neuro-ophthalmological evaluation before undergoing surgical or medical therapy. It is our responsibility, however, not only to examine the patients but also to provide our colleagues with information regarding the visual prognosis in such cases. We have the capability to determine, through both retrospective studies and prospective, controlled clinical trials, natural history compared with outcome after medical, surgical, or radiation therapy. Areas in which outcome assessment has already been applied include intracranial tumors, such as pituitary adenomas, suprasellar meningiomas, craniopharyngiomas, and optic nerve and chiasmal gliomas; disorders of the optic nerve, such as optic neuritis and ischemic optic neuropathy; and disorders of ocular motor nerves. I cannot overemphasize the importance of controlled clinical trials. Only with such trials can we hope to determine with a high degree of accuracy and a minimum of bias the effects of treatment on various disorders. I am hopeful that the future will see neuro-ophthalmologists continue to contribute to outcome assessment through controlled clinical trials.

■ Research Neuro-ophthalmology

As mentioned previously at the outset, the basis of neuro-ophthalmology has always been clinical observation of patients, leading to an understanding of pathophysiological mechanisms through clinicopathological correlation. In my opinion, it was W. Hoyt who first emphasized the importance of basic research and quantitative analysis to his fellows and students. Hoyt realized that to continue to contribute to our specialty, we must understand more than clinicopathological correlation. We must explore the physiological, genetic, and immunological bases for the diseases that we see, to more fully understand them. Many neuro-ophthalmologists now combine clinical work with laboratory investigations that include quantitative analysis of ocular motor function in normal and experimentally lesioned animals, assessment of histopathological and immunological changes in experimental optic neuritis, and an elucidation of the changes that occur in peripheral versus central nerves after injury that determine why regeneration occurs in peripheral nerves and not to any degree in central nerves. Recent breakthroughs in our understanding of the molecular genetics of various mitochondrial cytopathies of neuro-ophthalmological significance such as Leber's optic neuropathy, chronic progressive external ophthalmoplegia, the myoclonic epilepsy–lactic acidosis syndrome (MELAS), and the mitochondrial encephalopathy with ragged red fibers syndrome (MERRF), have already and will continue to attract the interests of neuro-ophthalmologists.

■ Therapeutic Neuro-ophthalmology

Many residents who have considered a career in neuro-ophthalmology have been put off because of their perception that the field is strong with respect to diagnosis but weak with respect to therapy. Nothing could be further from the truth. The tremendous improvements in the treatment of cerebrovascular disease and acute stroke, combined with improvements in neurosurgical and radiation therapy (including radiosurgery) for intracranial lesions, has resulted in an increase in the number of patients who would previously have died or survived with severe neurological deficits, but who now not only survive but have minor deficits. These often include difficulties in eye movements with consequent diplopia. Neuro-ophthalmologists are most capable of not only diagnosing but also treating surgically or with botulinum toxin (Oculinum) patients with ocular motor nerve pareses, skew deviation, internuclear ophthalmoplegia, and other gaze pareses. Neuro-ophthalmologists are also treating patients with blepharospasm, hemifacial spasm, and aberrant regeneration of the facial nerve with botulinum toxin. As new agents become available for the treatment of these and similar disorders, the neuro-ophthalmologist's role in both diagnosing and treating them will increase. Treatment of optic nerve disease, whether by medicine, surgery, or radiation therapy, will increasingly be the province of neuro-ophthalmologists. Dysthyroid optic neuropathy, for example, can be treated in a variety of ways. Neuro-ophthalmologists may elect to begin with a brief course of systemic corticosteroids. If patients do not respond to treatment, or the optic neuropathy worsens as steroids are tapered, neuro-ophthalmologists may elect to treat with radiation therapy (particularly if patients do not have significant proptosis or do not wish to undergo surgery) or with decompression surgery if patients have substantial proptosis. The role of optic nerve sheath surgery in the treatment of papilledema, anterior ischemic optic neuropathy, and other disorders of the optic nerve continues to be defined. It seems clear, however, that such surgery does have a place in the treatment of some optic nerve disorders and, again, is well within the province of neuro-ophthalmologists. Many neuro-ophthalmologists are operating on a regular basis with their colleagues in neurosurgery and otolaryngology on patients with tumors of the skull base that invade the cavernous sinus and orbit. I believe that this role in the team approach to such lesions will expand in the future.

In summary, I believe the future of neuro-ophthalmology is bright indeed. Our roles in diagnosis and teaching will continue, while our roles in outcome assessment, research, and therapy will expand. Join me in welcoming the future!

Management of Nonspecific Inflammatory and Lymphoid Orbital Lesions

John S. Kennerdell, M.D.

Management of lymphoid and noninfectious inflammatory lesions in the orbit is often difficult, and, therefore, there are a variety of opinions dealing with their management. Having had extensive experience with these entities, I have come to certain conclusions based on current knowledge. Of course, as information continues to accumulate on the etiology and course of these infiltrative disorders, recommendations will likely change. I describe current methods of management of these lesions and present some individual cases in which these principles were followed.

Nonspecific inflammatory lesions are comprised of a mixed cellular matrix including neurophils, plasma cells, histiocytes, macrophages, and some lymphocytes [1]. When a lesion is comprised predominantly of lymphocytes, however, it is referred to as a lymphoid lesion. The more benign forms have some other inflammatory cells, especially plasma cells, and have a tendency to form follicles. The intermediate types are comprised of benign-appearing lymphocytes with occasional plasma cells but no follicles. The more malignant types of lymphoid lesions show a variation of lymphoid cell type with irregular nuclei and staining.

Lymphoid lesions can be labeled more consistently with immunophenotyping. Lesions comprised mostly of either B cells or T cells are true lymphoma and are classified as malignant, whereas if the lesions are a mixture of B cells and T cells, they are usually benign. The lesions can be labeled with light chains such as alpha and kappa to differentiate further their makeup. Even with sophisticated cell markers providing accurate identification, however, it is not always possible to predict the future clinical course of orbital lymphoid lesions. It has been shown that benign, intermediate, and malignant lymphoid lesions are all associated with various percentages of future appearance of systemic lymphoid lesions [2].

Nonspecific orbital inflammatory lesions come in several forms. Some are targeted to one tissue in the orbit, causing myositis, perineuritis, periscleritis, or dacryoadenitis. These nonspecific lesions generally show a loose, mixed cellular infiltrate in the target tissue and begin most commonly in the acute form associated with pain and swelling. On computed tomography (CT) or magnetic resonance imaging (MRI), these lesions produce a thickening of the targeted tissue, sometimes with a ragged edge or extension into surrounding fat. More diffuse nonspecific inflammations that occur in the acute form can involve multiple orbital tissues and be quite extensive. They are also associated with swelling, erythema, and pain. In particular, the upper lid is often swollen. On CT or MRI they are more diffuse and conform to the contour of the eye or bony orbit. Nonspecific inflammatory lesions can begin in the subacute or chronic form and affect all of the tissues mentioned, which makes them more difficult to detect and manage.

Subacute and chronic forms are sometimes associated with formation of collagen followed by contracture of this scar tissue. These lesions are referred to as sclerosing, nonspecific orbital inflammation and are often very difficult to manage clinically [1].

Lymphoid lesions present as soft, nontender masses in the conjunctival area, eyelids, and all parts of the orbit. They can cause variable dysfunction, including ptosis, diplopia, and vision loss. If subconjunctival, they are pink or flesh colored. On CT or MRI they have smooth or irregular borders, conform to the contour of the bony orbit or globe, have usually uniform signal characteristics, and can involve the extraocular muscles, optic nerve, lacrimal gland and globe, as well as the orbital fat [3].

Management of these disorders demands early recognition and prompt intervention. Although some of the less serious acute nonspecific inflammatory lesions may resolve without treatment, such as myositis, the infiltrative lesions, whether nonspecific or lymphoid, do not resolve spontaneously in most cases. Therefore, an individualized management plan must be developed for these disorders based on knowledge of their likely course.

All patients with lymphoid lesions must have a biopsy prior to treatment, which can be performed with a fine needle technique. Fine needle aspiration, if successful (as it usually is with lymphoid lesions), can be extended to include immunophenotyping and DNA studies. This approach usually requires a second puncture, and in most cases does not need to be supplemented by open biopsy.

Superficial lesions, which are easily palpable, can be biopsied for tissue analysis. The same studies are carried out on the incisional biopsies to characterize the lesion as completely as possible. No lymphoid lesion should be treated on a presumptive basis.

Surprisingly, lymphoid lesions, although much more variable in their pathological presentation, are handled somewhat uniformly. In the past they have been treated with oral corticosteroids, which causes some reduction in the mass size but rarely accomplishes long-term control. In addition, patients are exposed to potential complications of long-term steroid therapy. Fortunately, these lymphoid lesions respond to moderate doses of radiation therapy (between 1,800 and 3,000 rads). I generally use approximately 2,500 rads for all benign or intermediate lesions and some lesions that are thought to be lymphomas if they are small and not associated with systemic disease. The radiation is delivered in 10 divided doses through a superolateral portal by radiotherapists experienced in working around the orbit with shielding of the eye [4, 5]. All patients, whether thought to have a malignant lymphoma or a benign lymphoid infiltrate, undergo systemic oncological studies, including abdominal CT scan, chest radiography, and bone marrow studies. The most common abnormality in asymptomatic patients with orbital lesions is a positive bone marrow aspirate. Therefore, bone marrow studies are an essential part of the initial oncological workup. Patients with known systemic disease are also treated with chemotherapeutic agents at the discretion of their oncologist.

Patients with bilateral orbital disease are usually found to have true lymphomas and are treated with higher doses of radiation therapy (e.g., 4,000 rads per orbit) supplemented by chemotherapy. If no systemic lymphoma is found, these patients must be watched carefully because of the higher incidence of systemic disease.

Patients who undergo treatment for lymphoid lesions of the orbit must be subject to follow-up for the rest of their lives. In my experience, there have been two orbital recurrences in 100 patients treated for orbital lymphoid lesions. Those two patients each were given another 2,500 rads radiation therapy and the lesions have resolved.

Management of nonspecific orbital inflammatory lesions is much more individualized. Patients presenting with acute inflammation involving a target organ are usually not biopsied but treated with prednisone. The dose for the average adult ranges between 80 and 100 mg per day in divided doses. Usually there is a prompt response in 24 to 48 hours, thus confirming the diagnosis. Patients must be tapered slowly off the prednisone because these acute lesions tend to recur and can change into subacute or chronic forms. Steroids are extended for at least four weeks, often up to 12 weeks with tapered dosage, to prevent recurrence. This prompt response is dramatic in that the swelling and pain disappear quickly and the function of the eye returns.

■ Case 1

A 66-year-old man was referred with left ptosis without discomfort for one month. His neuro-ophthalmic examination was normal except for a 2 mm left ptosis and a 3 mm left proptosis (Fig 1). On ultrasound and CT scan there was an infiltrative mass in the left superior orbit in the region of the levator and superior rectus (Fig 2). It was biopsied by fine needle aspiration and found to be a benign polyclonal lymphocytic infiltrate (Fig 3). The patient underwent a negative investigation for systemic lymphoma, and, after 2,500 rads of radiation therapy, the infiltrate resolved and has not recurred in one year of follow-up.

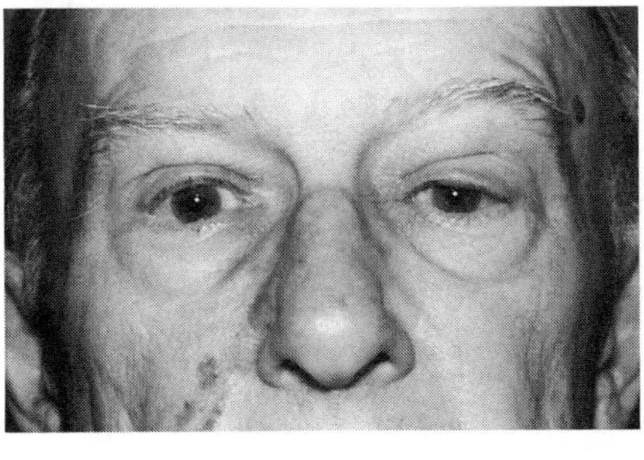

Figure 1 *A 66-year-old man with painless left proptosis and ptosis for one month.*

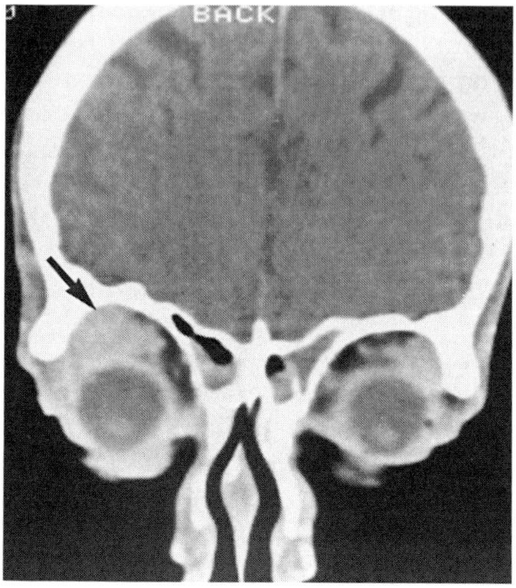

Figure 2 *Contrast-enhanced coronal computed tomographic scan reveals a mass* (arrow) *above the left globe that follows the contour of the superior orbit and the superior globe.*

■ Case 2

A 37-year-old man was referred with swelling of the right medial upper lid for two months. His neuro-ophthalmic examination was normal except for edema of the right upper lid and a palpable mass in the medial orbit. CT scan revealed a dense mass that molded to the globe but had somewhat irregular borders in the anterior medial orbit (Fig 4). The mass was removed through an anterior medial orbitotomy and proved to be a lymphoma (Fig 5). His systemic evaluation for lymphoma was negative and he was treated with 2,500 rads of radiation to the medial right orbit. One year after treatment he is free of disease, and CT shows resolution of the lesion (Fig 6). He will continue to

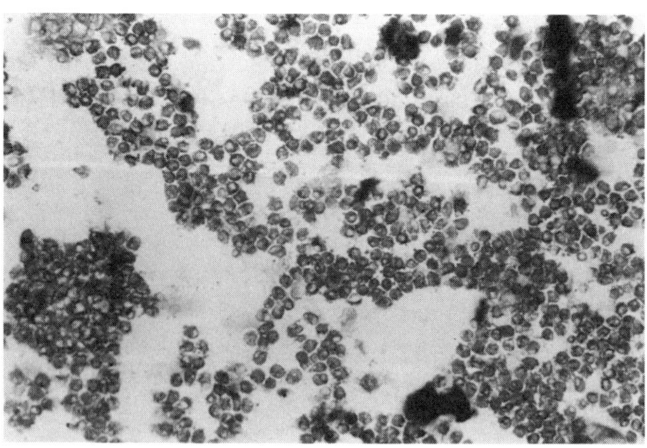

Figure 3 *Fine needle aspirate showing diffuse uniform population of small lymphocytes (Hematoxylin & Eosin, × 100).*

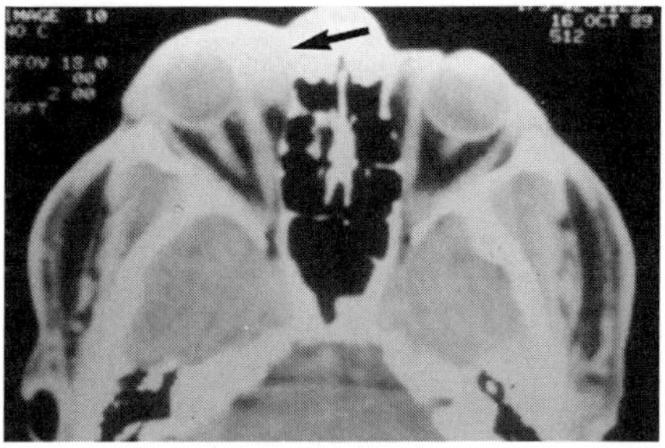

Figure 4 *Computed tomographic scan showing dense mass* (arrow) *molding to the right globe and extending out into the lid.*

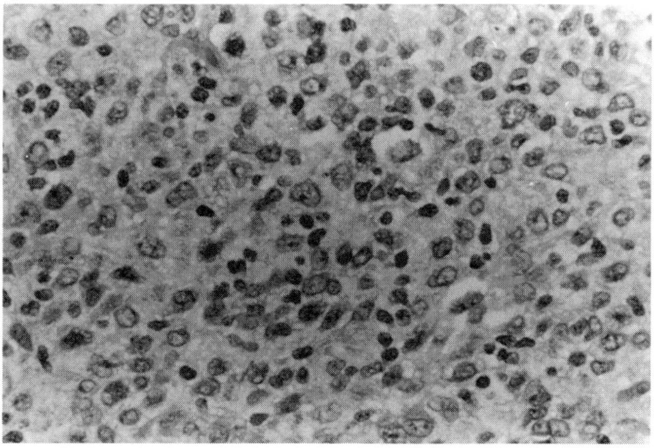

Figure 5 *Microscopic section showing cellular infiltrate composed of an equal number of small and large lymphocytes (Hematoxylin & Eosin, × 100).*

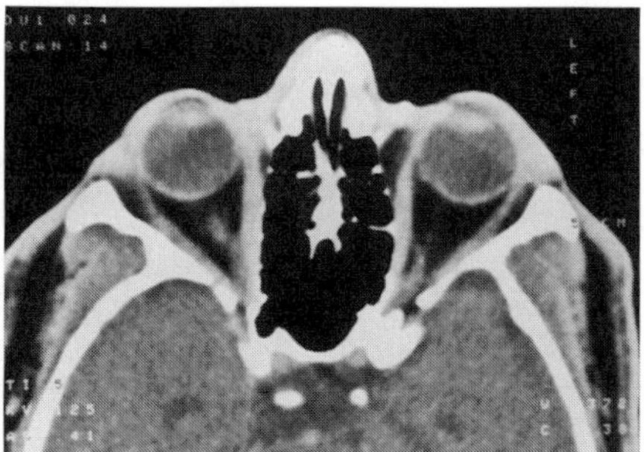

Figure 6 *Computed tomographic scan one year following treatment. No evidence of lesion in right medial orbit.*

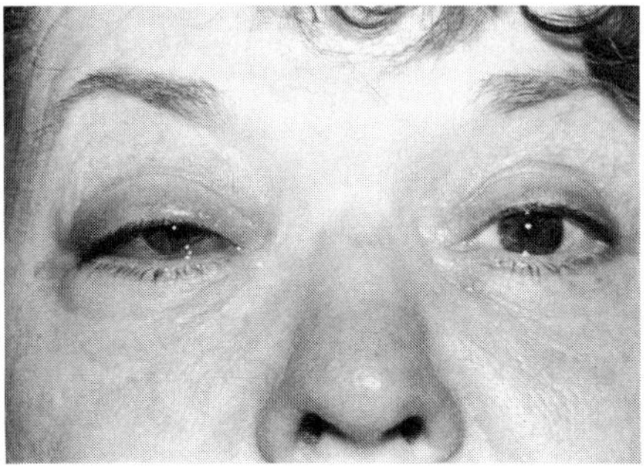

Figure 7 *A 57-year-old woman with edema and erythema of the right upper lid and conjunctiva caused by acute periscleritis.*

be followed up at six-month intervals and will have an orbital CT scan once each year.

■ Case 3

A 57-year-old woman was referred because of sudden onset of painful right periorbital swelling. There was no associated fever, and the patient had no previous history of infection. Her neuro-ophthalmic examination was normal except for 5 mm right proptosis with erythema and edema of the upper lid and conjunctiva with pain on eye movement (Fig 7). A CT scan revealed a periscleritic shaggy opacification (Fig 8). She was felt to have acute periscleritis and was placed on 80 mg of prednisone per day. This treatment promptly reversed the inflammatory process. Following cessation of prednisone, she has had no recurrence in six months.

■ Case 4

A 21-year-old man was referred with a long history of swelling of the right superior orbit associated with chronic pain and ptosis (Fig 9). An orbital mass

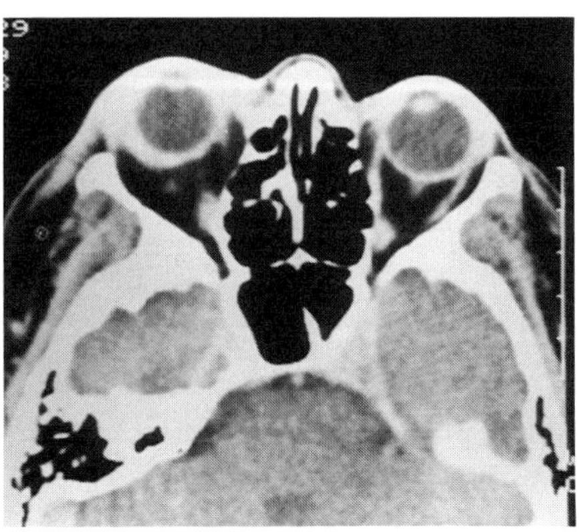

Figure 8 *Computed tomographic scan showing inflammation surrounding the right eye (concentrated anteriorly), representing periscleritis.*

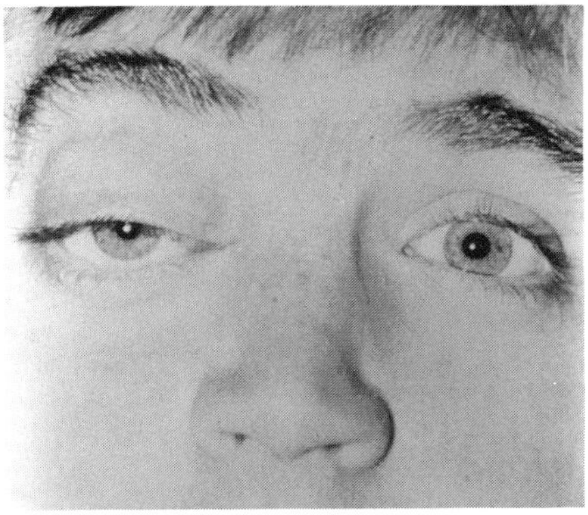

Figure 9 *A 21-year-old man with chronic right ptosis and proptosis accompanied by pain.*

was found on MRI in the superior extraconal space (Fig 10); it was biopsied and found to be sclerosing nonspecific orbital inflammation (Fig 11). There was partial response to high-dose oral prednisone, but right orbital pain and swelling recurred each time this medication was tapered. On referral, it was decided to excise the mass followed by radiation therapy to the superior orbit. This approach was carried out and he has done well postoperatively; pain and proptosis have been eliminated.

■ Discussion

Subacute or chronic nonspecific orbital lesions are much more difficult to treat and must be biopsied either by needle aspiration or by an incisional biopsy. Their treatment depends on the cellular infiltrate. If it is a soft, loose

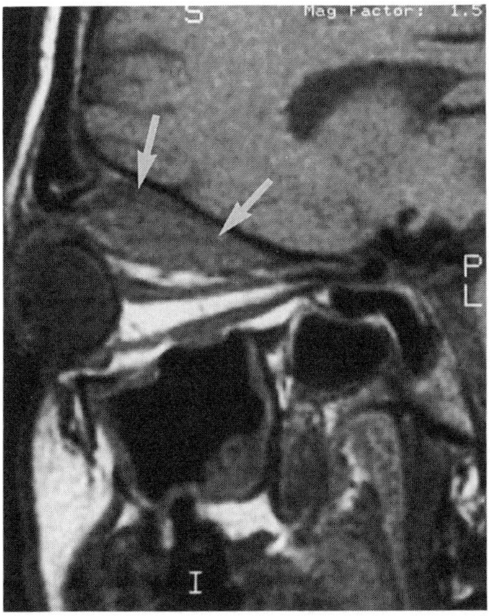

Figure 10 *T1-weighted sagittal magnetic resonance imaging demonstrates a mass* (arrows) *in the superior right orbit.*

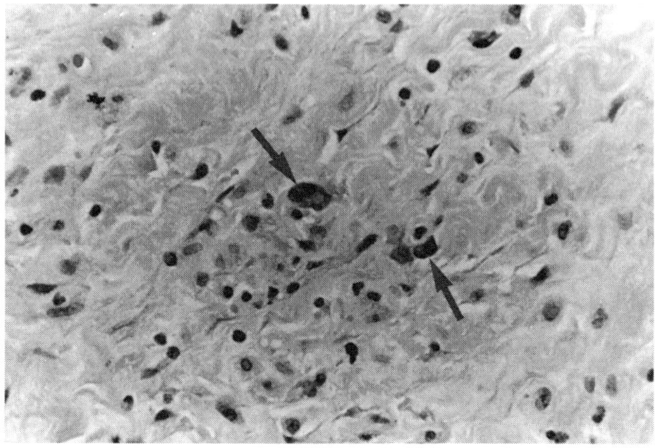

Figure 11 *Dense fibrosis with admixture of plasma cells* (arrows) *and small mature lymphocytes. The polymorphous composition of the cellular infiltrate is indicative of a benign process.*

infiltrate, it can respond to high-dose corticosteroids, similar to those used for acute nonspecific inflammation. Megadose steroids (e.g., 1,000 mg of methylprednisolone per day) are rarely necessary in treating nonspecific orbital inflammatory lesions. Chronic or subacute lesions, if not sclerosing, sometimes persist and recur. Generally, they respond to radiation therapy in a similar dosage to the lymphoid lesions (i.e., 2,000–3,000 rads in divided doses).

If the lesion is one in which collagen is laid down, causing sclerosis, it must be treated aggressively with a combination of high-dose oral corticosteroids and radiation therapy. The steroids inhibit the inflammatory process, although often not completely. Radiation therapy can further inhibit and in fact destroy the inflammatory process, but whatever collagen has been laid down will not shrink or disappear. Therefore, it is very important to be aggressive with these sclerosing lesions by performing a generous incisional biopsy in the earliest stage possible.

At times, sclerosing lesions are so resistant that chemotherapy must be used. Chemotherapy should be administered by an oncologist and should include methotrexate or cytoxan or both. Unfortunately, although these lesions can respond to both chemotherapeutic agents in combination with radiation and steroid therapy, the medications must be used on a long-term basis. In addition, it is occasionally necessary to repeat radiation therapy if patients suffer continued recurrences. Sometimes these lesions are so relentless that surgery to totally excise them is performed, followed by radiation therapy. Rarely, a modified exenteration is necessary for pain control. This procedure should be reserved for those patients in which vision has been destroyed by the lesion.

In summary, lymphoid and nonspecific orbital lesions may be difficult to manage and must be done so on a timely basis with a definite treatment plan. Diagnostic confusion can occur at any stage and there must be an accurate sampling of the lesion, which will provide a rational basis for therapy. These patients must be subjected to long-term follow-up because of a tendency for recurrence, and, in the case of lymphoid lesions, they must be reexamined by an oncologist because of the tendency for systemic involvement at a later date.

■ References

1. Kennerdell JS, Dresner SC. The non-specific orbital inflammatory syndromes. Surv Ophthalmol 1984;29:93–103
2. Knowles DM II, Jakobiec FA, Halper JP. Immunologic characterization of ocular adnexal lymphoid neoplasms. Am J Ophthalmol 1979;87:603–619
3. Yeo JH, Jakobiec FA, Abbot GF, Trokel SL. Combined clinical and computed tomographic diagnosis of orbital lymphoid tumors. Am J Ophthalmol 1982;94:235–245
4. Mittal BB, Deutsch M, Kennerdell JS, Johnson B. Paraocular lymphoid tumors. Radiology 1986;159:793–796
5. Gordon PS, Juillard GJF, Selch MT, et al. Orbital lymphomas and pseudolymphomas: treatment with radiation therapy. Radiology 1986;159:797–799

Ocular Lyme Borreliosis—1991

J. Lawton Smith, M.D.

The exploding medical literature now confronts practicing ophthalmologists with a dilemma that would cause even Sherlock Holmes to throw up his hands in despair—the subject of ocular and neurological involvement due to *Borrelia burgdorferi,* often simply called Lyme disease. First, we are dealing with a clinical entity unrecognized in this country before 1975. Second, the disease is due to an infectious agent that then defied recognition for over 6 years of intensive research before the *B. burgdorferi* spirochete was identified. Advances in knowledge of the disease since then have been rapid but so, also, has been spread of the disease.

The disease process is now known to involve virtually every human organ system and has mimicked syphilis, "the great imitator," not only clinically, but also serologically and pathologically. The disease has spread from initially being thought of as only endemic in New England to now having more than 14,000 cases reported from 46 states in the United States, and to a world-wide distribution; it has been reported from every continent except Antarctica. The disease was recognized clinically earlier in Europe with the sentinel skin lesion, erythema migrans, first reported in Sweden in 1909. Since recognition of the causative spirochete, it appears that the disease may be even more common in Europe than in the United States. As is true in any rapidly expanding field of medical knowledge, a number of controversies exist. For practicing ophthalmologists, these include the types and nature of ocular involvement in the disease; the frequency with which these occur; problems in serological diagnosis, including the detection of "seronegative" cases; the challenge of eradicating the organism in patients with chronic or late disease, particularly those previously treated with steroids; and finally, management of patients when symptoms recur frequently despite repeated courses of both oral and intravenous antibiotics. New information is appearing so rapidly concerning Lyme borreliosis that no final dogmatic opinion can be given at this time, and one should keep both an open mind and intellectual humility with regard to the subject.

Historical Background

In 1975, an outbreak of several cases of an illness initially diagnosed as juvenile rheumatoid arthritis occurred in the community of Old Lyme in southeastern Connecticut. A group of investigators from Yale University was called in to study these patients and the disease was named Lyme arthritis. A visiting dermatology fellow from Europe recognized that a sentinel sign of the disease was a specific cutaneous lesion known as erythema chronicum migrans (ECM), now called erythema migrans. This was a very important observation because this opened up over 6 decades of interesting clinical reports in the European literature. In October 1909, Afzelius at a dermatological meeting in Stockholm presented a patient with a lesion said to have resulted from a tick bite and called this "erythema chronicum migrans." The disease was thought to be strictly a cutaneous disorder until 1930, when Hellerstrom reported a patient with ECM and meningitis. In 1948, Lennhoff found spirochetes in these lesions, and this prompted Hollstrom in 1958 to report treating 77 of such patients with penicillin.

In 1955, Binder and associates [1] demonstrated the infectious nature of erythema migrans in a notable way. They took biopsy specimens from the active border of a clinically and histologically diagnostic erythema migrans lesion from a patient who had the lesion for 4 months. Portions of this lesion were then transplanted into a pocket of skin in the forearm of each of the 3 investigators. A typical erythema migrans lesion developed in 6 to 19 days in each physician. Tissue from one investigator's lesion was then transferred to his other arm, to the forearms of the other two investigators, and also into the forearm of a fourth person. Erythema migrans lesions formed at these new sites in all of them. The lesions disappeared within 2 to 4 days after treatment with 1.5 million units of penicillin. These findings were later confirmed by Sonck [2].

After realizing that Lyme arthritis was preceded by erythema migrans, and that erythema migrans was caused by a tick bite, a small tick (Ixodes dammini) was identified as the vector of the disease, and extracutaneous manifestations of the disease were promptly documented (with neurological, cardiac, testicular, and other involvements) and the name of the disease was changed from Lyme arthritis to Lyme disease.

An intense research effort began to identify the actual infectious organism, which was discovered by Burgdorfer and colleagues [3] in 1982, and the organism (Fig 1) was subsequently named *Borrelia burgdorferi* in his honor. All of Koch's postulates have since been confirmed with this organism.

■ Classification

The realization that Lyme spirochetosis bears many fundamental similarities to syphilis has given particularly helpful insights to the disease. For example, just as syphilis has been classically divided into three stages, so Lyme borreliosis may be considered as having primary, secondary, and tertiary stages. The first stage of Lyme disease begins with the tick bite in the skin followed by development of the characteristic skin lesion, erythema migrans. The tick is so small, however, that only 30% of patients with Lyme borreliosis recall having had a tick bite. Erythema migrans is a circular patch of spreading erythema, starting at the site of the tick bite, and this may gradually spread and become quite large. Some central clearing often occurs to give the ring-like

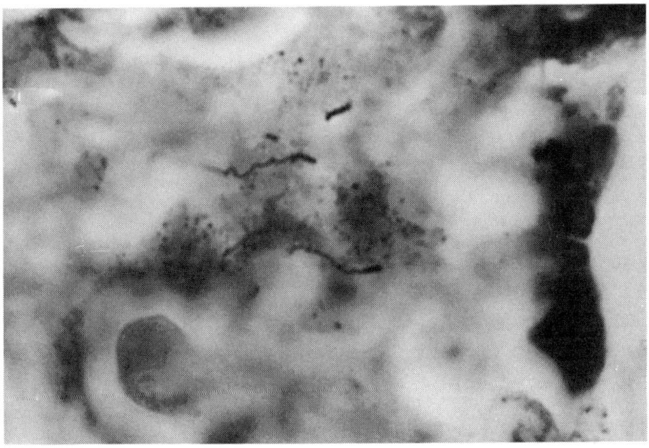

Figure 1 Borrelia burgdorferi *organisms provided through the courtesy of Dr Alan MacDonald. (Warthen Starry silver stain of placenta × 100.)*

lesion a "bull's-eye appearance" (Fig 2). Soon after the onset of this lesion, the organism disseminates throughout the blood stream and diffuse involvement occurs with symptoms mimicking a flu-like illness or infectious mononucleosis. Symptoms shortly after infection include conjunctivitis, pharyngitis, pneumonitis with dry cough and mild pleuritic pain, hepatosplenic tenderness, lymphadenopathy in neck and groin, and orchitis. Interestingly enough, if lumbar punctures are done during the primary stage because of headaches, stiff neck, and meningismus, they are consistently normal. An excellent clinical-pathological correlation of the various stages of Lyme borreliosis has been reported by Duray and Steere [4].

The second stage begins weeks to several months following initial infection and is usually evidenced by neurological or cardiovascular involvement. Duray and Steere [4] list the manifestations of stage two disease as follows: lymphocytoma cutis, iritis, panophthalmitis, meningitis, encephalitis, cranial neuritis (Bell's palsy), radiculoneuritis, myelitis, myocarditis, myositis, and fascitis. In

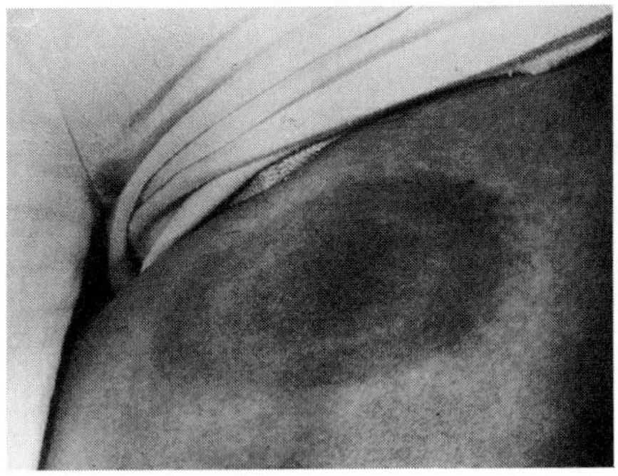

Figure 2 *Erythema migrans lesion showing "bull's-eye" ring. Provided by Dr Alan MacDonald.*

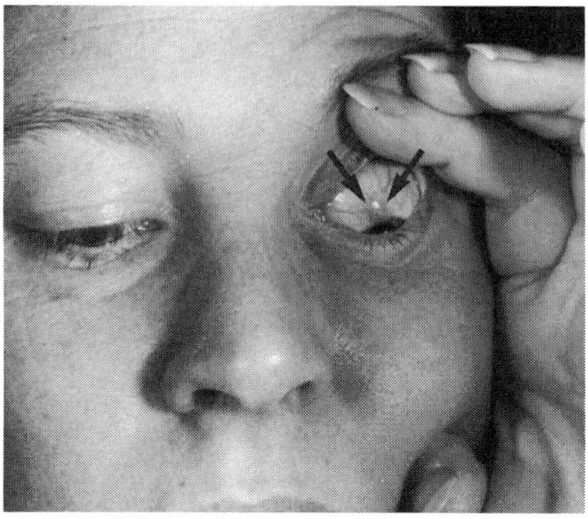

Figure 3 *Nodular episcleritis in Lyme disease. Provided by Dr Alan MacDonald.*

our experience the other forms of ocular involvement listed in Table 1 should be added to these signs of stage two disease, because significant ocular disease with Lyme borreliosis has been seen usually in late secondary or in early tertiary disease. Cranial or peripheral radiculoneuritides frequently occur in the second stage. The most common is a facial (Bell's) palsy. This palsy may be unilateral or bilateral, and it recurs frequently. Symptomatic meningitis occurs in approximately 15% of patients with Lyme disease. Lumbar puncture reveals a normal opening pressure with slightly cloudy fluid containing a lymphocytic pleocytosis. Bell's palsy is not only common with Lyme meningitis but is also frequently seen without meningitis. The triad of aseptic meningitis, cranial neuritis, and painful radiculitis has been emphasized in stage two disease.

The third stage of Lyme disease is the chronic phase, usually beginning months after onset and lasting for years. It is characterized by arthritis. This is intermittent oligoarthritis, most commonly involving the knee, but also frequently the wrist and shoulder. A variety of neurologic involvements, however, may dominate the third stage of the disease. These include multiple sclerosis–like syndromes, psychiatric disease, depressive reactions, chronic fatigue syndrome, an Alzheimer-like picture, amyotrophy, and a vasculitis simulating temporal arteritis [5]. Duray and Steere [4] list involvements in stage three Lyme disease as follows: arthritis-synovitis, vasculitis, myositis, fascitis, peripheral neuropathies, acrodermatitis chronica atrophicans, lymphocytoma cutis, linear scleroderma, ulnar fibrous nodules, and lichen sclerosus. Ackermann and co-workers [6] classify tertiary neuroborreliosis into: (1) progressive encephalomyelitis (predominantly spinal or predominantly cerebral), (2) peripheral neuropathy, and (3) latent neuroborreliosis. The clinical pictures of chronic fatigue, difficulty with memory and intellectual function, peripheral neuropathy, myopathies, neuropathies, plexopathies, focal encephalitis, demyelination–like illness, psychiatric syndromes, and lesions simulating "UBOs" (unidentified bright objects) on magnetic resonance imaging have incited both controversy and research.

The neurological manifestations of Lyme borreliosis will not be further mentioned in this review, but the major ones are listed in Table 2 [4–6].

Table 1 *Ocular Involvement in Lyme Borreliosis*

Lids
Erythema migrans (1° or 2°) on lids and periocular adnexae
Ptosis (neurological or protective)
Conjunctiva
Conjunctivitis—reported in 11% of patients with first stage disease
Episcleritis (see Fig 3)
Cornea
Acquired interstitial keratitis
Exposure keratitis with facial palsy
Impaired corneal reflex with V nerve involvement
Cogan's syndrome
Pupils
Horner's syndrome
Bilateral tonic pupils
Argyll Robertson–like pupils
Ocular motility
Diplopia due to III, IV, or VI nerve involvement
Uvea
Iritis
Cyclitis
Diffuse choroiditis with exudative retinal detachments
Vitreous
Chronic vitritis, unilateral or bilateral
Atypical pars planitis syndrome
Retina
Retinitis
Tractional retinal tears
Retinal vasculitis
Atypical Eales disease syndromes
Optic nerve
Optic neuritis (papillitis and retrobulbar neuritis)
Optic perineuritis
Papilledema with Lyme meningitis and atypical pseudotumor cerebri
Ischemic optic neuropathy
Big blind spot syndrome
Optic atrophy, secondary
Orbit
Orbital periostitis
Other
Panophthalmitis, cortical blindness

Table 2 *Neurological Involvement in Lyme Borreliosis*

Stage one Lyme disease
Headaches, meningismus
Stage two Lyme disease
Facial palsy, unilateral or bilateral
Aseptic meningitis
Bannwarth's syndrome
Cranial neuritis
Painful radiculitis
Meningopolyneuritis
Encephalitis
Radiculoneuritis
Myelitis
Stage three Lyme disease
Progressive encephalomyelitis
Mostly spinal (multiple sclerosis–like)
Mostly cerebral (multifocal encephalitis or psychosis)
Peripheral polyneuritis (associated with acrodermatitis chronica atrophicans)
Latent neuroborreliosis
Chronic fatigue
Difficulty with memory and intellectual function
Myopathies
Neuropathies, plexopathies
Psychiatric disorders

■ Ocular Lyme Borreliosis

Ocular involvement in Lyme borreliosis has received gradually increasing interest. Steere and associates [7] in 1985 reported a 45-year-old woman in whom a fulminating unilateral iritis and vitritis developed 4 weeks after onset of erythema migrans, which, despite massive doses of intravenous methicillin sodium and gentamicin, progressed to lensectomy and vitrectomy. Examination of the surgical specimen with silver stains revealed spirochetes morphologically compatible with Lyme disease spirochetes. Serial serum antibody titers were immunoglobulin M (IgM) 1:64 and IgG 1:512. Two months later, the IgG titer had decreased to 1:64, and 7 months later, neither specific IgG nor IgM antibody was found.

Wu and colleagues [8] in 1986 reported a 7-year-old boy who was in good health until 2 months before admission when he developed a red skin lesion on the cheek after an insect bite. Three days later, a generalized maculopapular rash, fever of 40°C, headaches, nausea, and vomiting appeared. Oral penicillin therapy was given for 3 days but was discontinued when his symptoms improved. Several weeks later, the boy was lethargic, had pain in wrists and elbow, and was taken to an ophthalmologist because of red eyes. Bilateral "papilledema" prompted hospitalization. The subsequent course was consistent with bilateral optic neuritis with good vision (or optic perineuritis), in that he developed cecocentral scotomas in both eyes, and lumbar puncture revealed an opening pressure of 170 mm with 14 leukocytes/mm^3. CT of the brain was normal. A blood titer for *B. burgdorferi* was positive at 1:256, and he responded promptly to a course of intravenous penicillin. One year later, vision was 20/20 in both eyes and he had no complaints.

Although there has been controversy about the incidence and types of ocular involvements in Lyme borreliosis, it is evident that ocular involvement is much more common in Lyme borreliosis than is commonly appreciated (see Table 1). A few illustrative cases [9, 10] will be cited to show the typical ocular features as noted in the Bascom Palmer Eye Institute experience.

■ Case Reports

Case 1 (R. C.)

A 25-year-old man was seen in July 1988 with blurred vision. Three years earlier after a "viral infection" he developed bilateral facial palsies that promptly improved with steroids. One year later, and again in 1987, he had recurrences of "Bell's palsy" on the left, which responded to steroids. Six weeks prior to the first visit, he developed blurred vision in the right eye. His ophthalmologist noted iritis and prescribed topical steroids and cycloplegics. A thorough rheumatological evaluation gave negative results except for a positive serum Lyme enzyme-linked immunosorbent assay (ELISA) test. Past history revealed unexplained arthritis in one knee for 2 months, occasional palpitations, and he remembered a tick bite while hunting in the Everglades and that he had camped at Cape Cod at ages 11 and 14.

Examination revealed corrected vision of 20/15 − 2, right eye and 20/30 + 2, left eye. Mild aberrant regeneration of the left VII nerve was evident. Biomicroscopy revealed clear anterior chambers but 2+ cells in the vitreous of both eyes. Whitish deposits were seen in the preretinal space, as well as a retinal tear in the left eye with white exudate on an attached flap.

Extensive hematological studies were normal, as were chest radiographs and magnetic resonance imaging of the head. Lumbar puncture revealed 9 white cells/mm^3, but was otherwise normal. Serum Lyme indirect fluorescent antibody test (IFA) IgG and IgM was negative, but Lyme ELISA was again positive (1.81). (Microbiology Reference Laboratory, Cypress, CA, reports Lyme ELISA < 0.85 as negative, 0.85–1.25 as borderline, and > 1.25 as positive.) Serum Western blot test was also positive for Lyme disease. The Lyme ELISA was repeated and confirmed as positive at a third laboratory.

Topical steroids and cycloplegics, oral doxycycline, and erythromycin were given but without improvement. Bilateral iridocyclitis developed and the vitritis worsened in both eyes. Intravenous ceftriaxone sodium (2 g/day) and intravenous aqueous penicillin G (12 million units/day) were given. Two weeks later, the inflammation was markedly reduced and acuity was 20/15 in both eyes. After a 1-month course of intravenous antibiotics, oral tetracycline was started (1 g/day). After his eyes had been quiet for 9 months, the tetracycline was tapered. Within 1 month, however, iritis and vitritis recurred with posterior synechiae (Fig 4). Cefuroxime therapy (500 mg/day) resulted again in improvement, and the patient was maintained on this drug orally. In September 1989, he returned with a recurrence of blurred vision. Vision was 20/30, right eye and 20/60, left. Minimal inflammation was present but vitreous de-

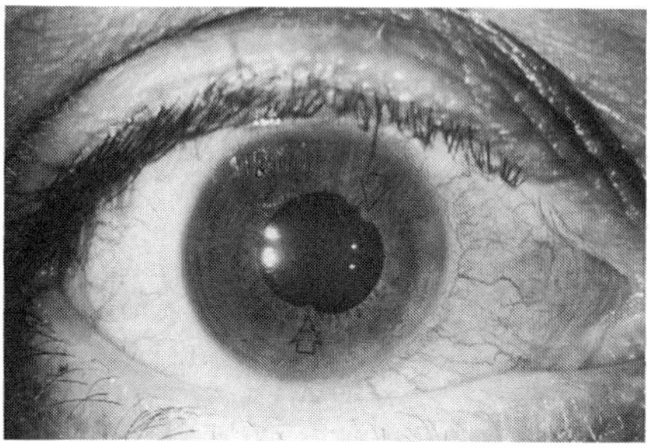

Figure 4 *Case 1. Koeppe nodules and posterior synechiae.*

posits (Fig 5) and snow banking inferiorly and small tufts of retinal neovascularization were seen just off the disc in both eyes. Cystoid macular edema was present in the left eye, and fluorescein angiography showed retinal vasculitis in both eyes. Oral tetracycline (250 mg, 4 times a day) was started, and 2 weeks later his condition was unchanged. Twenty mg subtenons Kenalog (Westwood–Squibb, Buffalo, NY) was given on the left; no oral steroids were given and the patient was continued on tetracycline. On October 10, 1989, the patient was notably improved; vision was 20/25 − 2, right and 20/40 + 2, left. Repeat fluorescein angiography documented marked improvement of the retinal vasculitis.

The patient was maintained on oral tetracycline (1 gm/day) thereafter. Follow-up in July 1990 revealed vision of 20/20 − for both eyes, quiet anterior segments, 1+ old vitreous cells in both eyes, normal discs, and the patient was comfortable.

Comment The diagnosis of late Lyme borreliosis was made in this 27-year-old man on the basis of the following criteria: (1) he was an outdoorsman who remembered a definite tick bite, (2) exposure to an endemic area, (3) arthralgias, (4) palpitations, (5) three episodes of recurrent Bell's palsy. In addition, (6) extensive medical and rheumatological investigation for other etiologic causes of his chronic recurrent ocular inflammatory disease were negative. (7) He had definitely positive serum ELISA tests for Lyme borreliosis on more than 3 occasions in 3 different laboratories and also had a positive serum Western blot for this disease. Although he had been treated with steroids in the

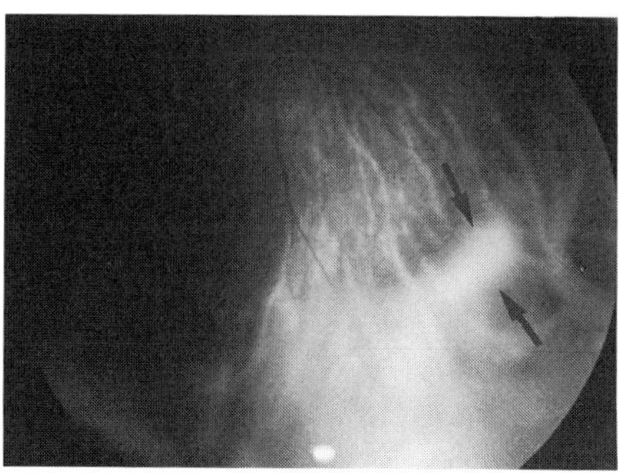

Figure 5 *Case 1. Preretinal "snowball" in vitreous.*

past, (8) he showed dramatic responses to intravenous antibiotics on repeated occasions. (9) There was no other evident disease on over 2 years' follow-up. Eye manifestations in this patient were his chief complaint throughout, with chronic bilateral recurrent vitritis as the predominant feature, but also including iritis, tractional retinal tear, cystoid macular edema, and retinal vasculitis.

Case 2 (L. R.)

An 11-year-old girl from Wisconsin, a highly endemic area for Lyme borreliosis, developed red painful eyes in 1988. She was found to have chronic pars planitis syndrome, which was atypical in association with iritis and posterior synechiae. Although Lyme IFA was normal on 2 occasions, serum Lyme ELISA was strongly positive (2.1; normal, <0.85, and borderline, 0.85–1.25) and the patient had a dramatic response to intravenous Rocephin (Roche Laboratories, Nutley, NJ) therapy. This may be called the Lyme pars planitis syndrome. Culbertson has emphasized this constellation of findings as atypical for the usual cases of pars planitis, so it may be referred to as Culbertson's triad (bilateral vitritis/pars planitis, with iritis and posterior synechiae) and should make ophthalmologists think immediately of Lyme borreliosis.

Case 3 (J. P.)

This 28-year-old Haitian man was seen in 1988 with a chief complaint of decreasing vision for 1 year. He had moved to Miami from Haiti 6 years earlier, with no complaints until 1 year prior to presentation when he developed ocular redness, mild pain, and photophobia, followed by progressive bilateral loss of vision. He had been seen in New Jersey and treated for "iritis" with topical steroids and cycloplegics, but without improvement.

Examination in January 1988 revealed a vision of finger counting in the right eye and 20/400 in the left eye. Slit lamp examination revealed 1+ cells and flare, pigmented keratic precipitates, posterior synechiae, and 2+ vitreous cells in both eyes. The fundi were difficult to visualize because of the dense bilateral vitritis. Results of a neurological examination were normal.

Laboratory findings revealed a sedimentation rate of 105 mm/hr, with a white blood cell count of 15,000/mm^3; 82% were neutrophils. Rheumatoid factor, antinuclear antibody, cryoglobulins, Raji cell assay, C3 and C4 complement components, angiotensin converting enzyme, human immunodeficiency virus ELISA, rapid plasma reagin (RPR), fluorescent treponemal antibody-absorption (FTA-ABS), treponema pallidium immobilization (TPI), and treponema pallidium hemagglutination (TPHA) were normal. An intermediate strength tuberculin skin test revealed 10 mm induration. Chest radiograph was normal. Lyme IFA IgG was less than 1:16, but IgM was positive at 1:320; this test was confirmed positive at another laboratory. Lumbar puncture revealed an opening pressure of 230 mm water, with 30/mm^3 white blood cells (75% lymphocytes, 25% immature neutrophils), 31 mg% protein, 59 mg% glucose, and nonreactive VDRL. Cultures for bacteria, fungi, and acid-fast organisms were negative.

The patient was treated with intravenous Rocephin (2 gm/day), and 3 days later 12 million units/day of aqueous penicillin G was added. Intravenous antibiotics were given for 7 days, followed by 2 gm/day of oral tetracycline for 3 weeks. Visual acuity improved to 20/70 in the right eye and 20/80 in the left eye, and marked clearing of the vitritis was evident.

The patient was then lost to follow-up for 1 year, but then returned with a blind phthisical right eye and left eye vision down to finger counting. The left eye showed anterior uveitis with posterior synechiae and a dense secondary cataract. After further antibiotic therapy, a vitrectomy/lensectomy was performed on the left eye in October 1990. Studies at that time revealed blood IgG was 1,550 (normal, 800–1,800) and serum Lyme ELISA was 1.45 (reference 0–0.99). The patient's vitreous IgG level was 102, and vitreous Lyme ELISA was 0.08. The left eye vision improved to 20/200, and ophthalmoscopy showed a pale optic disc, narrow vessels, and chorioretinal scarring.

Comment A 28-year-old Haitian man developed chronic bilateral anterior uveitis and vitritis in 1987. Extensive investigation repeatedly revealed only positive serum Lyme IgM titers, and he had a dramatic visual improvement following a course of intravenous antibiotic therapy. The inflammation recurred when the patient was lost to follow-up, but after vitrectomy/lensectomy, vision in the left eye improved from finger counting to 20/200.

Case 4 (L. C.)

In 1975 a 26-year-old woman presented with an erythematous lesion on her right ankle. Within a few weeks, she had a severe flu-like illness, followed by bilateral facial palsies. In early 1984 she developed blurred vision and floaters and was found to have pars planitis. During the next 2 years, multiple recurrences of ocular inflammation were treated with steroids with only moderate response.

In 1988 she again developed a right VII nerve palsy. Visual acuity was 20/70 in the right eye and 20/60 in the left eye. Several large keratic precipitates, moderate cells and flare, and posterior synechiae were present. Prominent vitritis (Fig 6) with snowbanked exudates was noted. An extensive medical investigation was negative except for a Lyme IFA IgG of 1:128 and a Lyme ELISA of 1.7. A 10-day course of intravenous ceftriaxone sodium without steroids resulted in prompt improvement. A later recurrence again responded to intravenous ceftriaxone. The left eye subsequently required vitrectomy; postoperative acuity was 20/40, and the eye remained quiet thereafter.

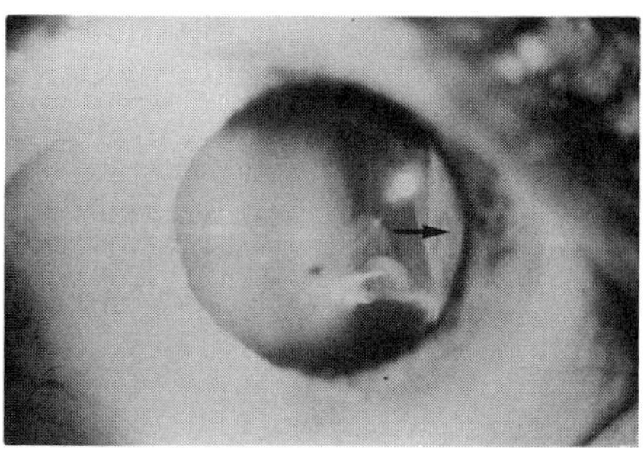

Figure 6 *Case 4. Chronic vitreous opacification with dense bands* (arrow).

■ Vitreous Organisms in Experimental Animal Studies

Although there is still a definite need for an appropriate animal model to study ocular and neurological manifestations of Lyme borreliosis, some investigations using rabbits and hamsters have provided useful background information. Because of the frequent finding of vitritis in patients with historical and serological evidences of prior infection with *B. burgdorferi*, a particularly interesting report by Duray and Johnson [11] is of interest. This report concerned the histopathology of Syrian hamsters experimentally infected with *B. burgdorferi.* Seven hamsters inoculated intraperitoneally with 100,000,000 organisms were examined for 1 to 9 months. At necropsy all animals appeared clinically well. None showed significant histological abnormalities in many tissues examined. The following statements are pertinent, however; "Whole eye sections showed occasional mononuclear phagocytic cells in the ocular vitreous fluid of animals 3 and 4. Spirochetes were particularly easy to visualize in the vitreous of the eyes of animals 4 and K1-1. Here the morphology of the organisms was strikingly similar to that seen in the maintenance culture controls. Ocular spirochetes were in greater numbers in the vitreous relative to the numbers seen in the liver, spleen, or kidneys." The authors further commented "The spirochetes' attraction for the eye may be related to the viscosity of the vitreous as well as the glucose and electrolyte content [11]. Ocular vitreous viscosity qualitatively is similar to that provided by adding 0.1% agarose to BSK media." This experimental observation of the presence of intact *B. burgdorferi* spirochetes in the vitreous humor unaccompanied by other than occasional mononuclear cells in animals inoculated intraperitoneally certainly is consistent with the finding of vitritis in the eyes of some patients with late secondary or early third-stage Lyme borreliosis and merits further study.

■ Serological Tests

Spirochetal Serological Similarities

Current controversies about the serological criteria for the diagnosis of Lyme borreliosis immediately bring to mind, to anyone familiar with the history of syphilis, the statement of Solomon that "there is no new thing under the sun." To approach the subject of seronegative neuroocular Lyme borreliosis, it would be helpful to briefly review the development of this concept regarding *B. burgdorferi*'s amazingly comparable elder brother, the "gold standard" spirochete, *Treponema pallidum.*

Syphilis Serology Space does not allow nor is the author qualified to cover in depth the laboratory aspects of this subject, but the following may be helpful to clinicians. Holmes' text [12] contains references that will help the reader who desires to pursue the subject further.

First, why are serological tests so important for the diagnosis of spirochetal disease? Tables 3 and 4 may illustrate this point. It should be recalled that no one has ever been able to culture virulent *T. pallidum* in vitro, and the only way the organism can be definitively recovered from an infected host is by

Table 3 *Ways to Diagnose Syphilis*

Clinical history and examination
Dark-field microscopy
Serological tests
Histopathology
Passive transfer

passive transfer to animals. The latter has been classically done by intratesticular inoculation into rabbits, an obviously laborious procedure. Fortunately, *B. burgdorferi* has been grown on artificial media in vitro but to date this has been not only tedious but a very low-yield procedure. The difficulties involved in growing *B. burgdorferi* notwithstanding, the growth of the organism from patients has been accomplished in several very important studies [13–15]. Dark-field microscopy is much more practical when dealing with chancres and moist mucous membrane syphilitic lesions teeming with organisms than with later lesions of either syphilis or Lyme borreliosis, because it requires at least 10^4 treponemes per mm of transudate to be detected [16]. Histopathology of both diseases not only reveals similar-appearing histological lesions but requires exhaustive searches for spirochetes under silver stains that are not specific in any way, or requires special techniques (fluorescent microscopy), restricting their use in practice to investigational laboratories. The polymerase chain reaction holds great promise for the diagnosis of syphilis [17], but is not as yet commercially available.

Lyme Borreliosis Serology Just as fluorescent antibody techniques have been widely applied in both serological and tissue diagnosis of syphilis, as well as other infectious diseases, so these techniques were applied early on in the serological investigations of patients with Lyme disease. The first test investigated in our department was the Lyme IFA IgG and IgM test. More commonly employed at this time, however, is the ELISA test for *B. burgdorferi,* because this test has been automated and can be more readily performed on large numbers of samples. Space does not allow a description of these procedures, which are now commonly performed in this country. A brief summary of serological testing for Lyme borreliosis done at the Bascom Palmer Eye Institute is of interest, however, particularly when one compares the finding of the test results in Lyme borreliosis with those of ocular syphilis.

Why should we be concerned about syphilis serology in a chapter devoted to ocular Lyme borreliosis? Shortly after the description of *B. burgdorferi* as

Table 4 *Ways to Diagnose Lyme Borreliosis*

Clinical history and examination
Serological tests
Histopathology
Culture

the causative agent for Lyme disease, cross-reactivity between *T. pallidum* and *B. burgdorferi* was demonstrated in both immunofluorescent and ELISA [18].

Because of the known high incidence of reactive FTA-ABS tests in the clinic population at Bascom Palmer Eye Institute [19], and to study the incidence of seroreactivity for Lyme disease in a nonendemic area, serological tests for both Lyme borreliosis and for syphilis were performed on 75 patients seen at the Bascom Palmer Institute in one week in late March 1988 [20]. Thirty-five sera were from preoperative cataract patients; 15 sera were from follow-up patients in the neuro-ophthalmic outpatient clinic; and 25 sera were from consecutive/consenting patients coming to the eye triage/emergency clinic during 2 days of that period. Testing revealed an 8% incidence of syphilis and a 3% incidence of Lyme borreliosis in this area. It merits emphasis that the most common cause for a high-titered serological response for Lyme borreliosis in this group was a prior *T. pallidum* infection. The importance of getting VDRL, FTA-ABS, Lyme IFA, and Lyme ELISA tests in all suspected cases was emphasized.

A second report [21] extended this study by summarizing data on 641 sera drawn between September 1987 and January 1990. Of the 641 sera tested, 10% showed reactive RPR tests and 22% showed reactive FTA-ABS tests. Lyme IFA IgG titers were 1:64 or more in 17% of the sera, and Lyme ELISA tests were more than 1.25 in 15% of the sera. Our experience correlated with previous reports that serum RPR or VDRL tests are nonreactive in Lyme borreliosis, but that false-positive FTA-ABS tests can occur in Lyme borreliosis. The latter phenomenon is not common but does occur, and appears to have occurred in approximately 12 cases in nearly 1,000 sera studied to date. False-positive FTA-ABS tests have been described with lupus erythematosus, both systemic and discoid varieties, and may also cause false-positive (MHA-TP) tests.

False-Positive Serum FTA-ABS Tests in Lyme Borreliosis The FTA-ABS test is the most commonly employed treponemal test in the United States for confirmation of the diagnosis of syphilis. The specificity of this test has been reported to be between 92 to 99%. It is important, however, for clinicians to understand the interrelationships between the serological tests for these two major spirochetal diseases—syphilis, caused by *T. pallidum,* and Lyme borreliosis, caused by *B. burgdorferi.* After the identification of *B. burgdorferi* as the causative agent of Lyme borreliosis, it was recognized that cross-reactivity between *T. pallidum* and *B. burgdorferi* was frequently seen in both IFA and ELISA tests when sera from patients with Lyme disease or syphilis were tested. However, a definitive study by Hunter and associates [18] from the Centers for Disease Control in 1986 revealed that when 40 sera from patients with Lyme disease were examined in the FTA-ABS test with *T. pallidum* antigen, 9 (22.5%) showed reactive tests. None of the sera tested from patients with Lyme disease showed reactive RPR or MHA-TP tests for syphilis. The authors pointed out, however, that the MHA-TP test is known to be less sensitive than the FTA-ABS test, especially for detecting primary syphilis. An important point is that 9 of 40 sera were reactive at the 1:5 dilution on the FTA-ABS test. Only 1 serum was reactive at 1:10 dilution. Hunter and colleagues [18] point out that one could usually differentiate between *T. pallidum* and *B. burgdorferi* serologically by studying serial titers and finding a higher titer with the specific organism. The point to the practitioner, however, is that when one orders a serum FTA-ABS test, it is *routinely* run at a 1:5 dilution. Other dilutions are not available except on a research basis. There is no question that one can encounter false-positive serum FTA-ABS test results in patients with Lyme disease.

The interrelationships between serological responses to syphilis and Lyme disease are so important that the clinician is advised to always request studies for both diseases whenever the diagnosis of either one is considered. A Lyme/treponemal panel is commonly used in our department, which includes a serum RPR, FTA-ABS, Lyme IFA IgG and IgM, and Lyme ELISA test. We have found Microbiology Reference Laboratory (Cypress, CA) to be a reliable facility and the least expensive provider of this panel. As stated previously, the incidence of syphilis is 8% in our patient population in Miami and the incidence of Lyme disease appears to be 3% in this institution [20]. The highest titers for Lyme disease were found in patients who had unequivocal serological evidence for syphilis. A more recent review of 641 sera studied in this department between September 1987 and January 1990 showed that of all sera tested, 10% showed reactive RPR tests and 22% showed reactive FTA-ABS tests. We have seen only approximately 2 reactive RPR tests in patients with nonreactive FTA-ABS tests in the past 1,000 or so sera studied and both were borderline or of low titer (1 dilution), and the incidence of biological false-positive RPR tests is therefore probably no higher in this group than in the normal population. At this point, we conclude that the serum RPR or VDRL test should be negative in patients with Lyme disease, which is a very helpful differentiating point in separating patients with Lyme borreliosis from those with syphilis. It should be pointed out that a positive serum FTA-ABS test should certainly make one suspicious of syphilis in the first place, and that further serological testing and careful historical investigation is in order.

■ "Seronegative" Late Ocular and Neurosyphilis

The frequency with which patients are seen with clinical signs of late ocular and neurosyphilis but with nonreactive or negative routine serum VDRL or RPR tests prompted the author to publish *Spirochetes in Late Seronegative Syphilis, Penicillin Notwithstanding* in 1969 [22]. The definition of seronegative syphilis used was (1) a patient showing clinical signs or symptoms of late syphilis; (2) exclusion of other etiological causes by appropriate study; (3) a nonreactive serum reagin test (VDRL or RPR); (4) a reactive specific or treponemal test (TPI or FTA-ABS); and/or (5) demonstration of the spirochete. The demonstration of treponemes in various tissues and body fluids in patients despite treatment with significant courses of penicillin was shown at that time and has been confirmed in more than 11 different laboratories around the world. The point is that when seeing a patient with, for example, light-near dissociation of the pupils, pale optic discs, old granulomatous chorioretinitic scars in the fundi, or with an unexplained recurrent iridocyclitis, one should not rely on the finding of a nonreactive or negative serum VDRL test to exclude the possibility that the disease process was due to syphilis, but should obtain an FTA-ABS or TPI test in such a patient.

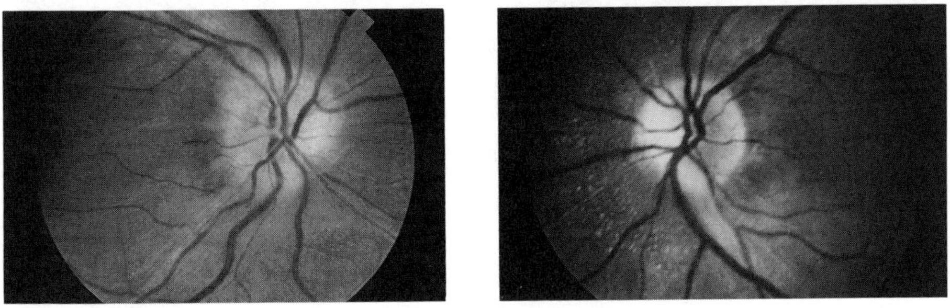

A B

Figure 7 *Case 5. Right optic disc (A) is swollen, whereas left fundus (B) reveals disc swelling and white deposits due to neuroretinitis.*

■ "Seronegative" Late Ocular or Neurological Lyme Borreliosis

Exactly the same situation prevails today with Lyme borreliosis as was confronted with syphilis over 40 years ago when the TPI test was described. The criteria for the diagnosis of "seronegative" late Lyme borreliosis might be (1) a patient with a history or physical findings suspicious for Lyme borreliosis; (2) exclusion of other etiological causes by appropriate investigation; (3) a nonreactive or negative result on a routine serum Lyme IFA or ELISA test; (4) a positive test on further testing (Western blot, lymphocyte stimulation assay, polymerase chain reaction, or urine antigen study); (5) definitive response to appropriate antibiotic therapy as a supporting criterion; and (6) demonstration of the spirochete by histopathological techniques or recovery of the *B. burgdorferi* organism by culture.

There appears to be no question that some cases of "seronegative" Lyme disease exist [23] or that some cases of late latent Lyme borreliosis exist [5]. What is controversial is the frequency with which these occur and the magnitude of this problem in practice.

Case 5 (T. P.)

A healthy 28-year-old man had close exposure to deer working at an outdoor site in Minnesota in June 1988. Shortly thereafter, he developed progressively incapacitating fatigue, arthralgias, and abdominal and chest pain with such weakness that within 6 months he went from benchpressing 410 lbs and running 5 miles in less than 30 minutes, to requiring 2 to 3 nurses to help him out of a wheelchair. He developed bilateral recurrent optic neuritis with pain on motion of the globe (Fig 7). The patient had a mild leukocytic pleocytosis with slight elevation of spinal fluid protein, confirmed on 2 subsequent lumbar punctures. Magnetic resonance imaging showed only a few periventricular white matter hypodense lesions or "UBOs." The predominant part of his illness was recurrent optic nerve disease, which left him with constricted visual fields and pale discs (Fig 8). He had only transient responses to repeated

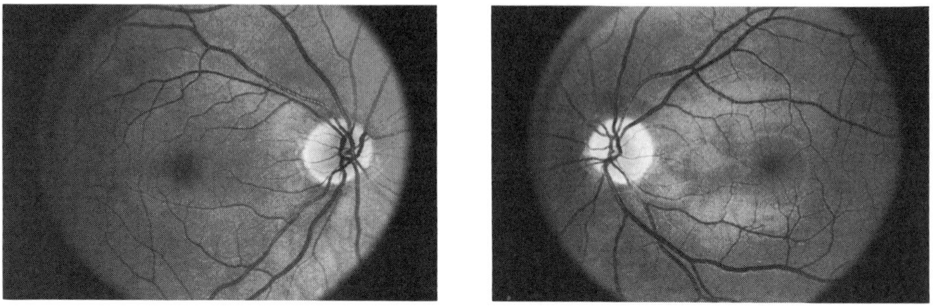

A B

Figure 8 *Case 5. Appearance of fundi 17 months later shows bilateral optic atrophy. A ghost "high-water mark" remains on nasal side of right disc (A) denoting extent of previous swelling. A glial remnant remains of the nasal aspect of left disc (B) as a residual sign of previous inflammation.*

courses of oral and intravenous antibiotic therapy. Extensive investigations for other etiological causes were negative. However, the patient had two borderline Lyme ELISA tests and showed a positive Lyme lymphocyte antigen stimulation test. It was determined that he had optic atrophy, in both eyes, secondary to bilateral neuroretinitis caused by Lyme borreliosis; he was seronegative but had a positive lymphocyte antigen stimulation test.

■ Office Workup

History

The most important part of the workup for ophthalmologists is to have a high index of suspicion for both Lyme borreliosis and syphilis, and to ask the right questions in the right way and at the right time. The following questions should be explored with any patient with uveitis, cranial neuropathy, or unexplained neuro-ophthalmologic symptoms.

Geographic Questions What part of the country were you born in? How long did you live there? What parts of the country have you visited? When? If a patient is from New England (Connecticut, New York, Massachusetts, Vermont, Pennsylvania, New Jersey), from the upper midwest (Wisconsin, Minnesota), from the far Pacific west coast, or from Texas, Missouri, or Florida, these are the most endemic areas for Lyme disease.

Exposure Questions Are you an outdoorsperson, or do you like camping out? What animals have you been exposed to? Ticks, deer, mice, cattle, dogs? Have you had any sick pets (e.g., dogs with lameness or arthritis)? Do you recall a tick bite? Have you had a skin lesion consistent with erythema migrans (show them a picture) at any time?

Early Lyme Disease Questions Did you have a flu-like illness before your eye problem began? What were your symptoms? Did you run a fever then?

Were you treated with antibiotics, and if so, what drug was used, in what dosage, and for how long? What was your response?

Other Lyme Disease Questions Have you ever had a Bell's palsy? Have you ever had aseptic meningitis? Have you had any type of arthritis? Have you noted a problem with chronic fatigue? Any change in memory?

Treatment Questions Have you been treated with steroids? If so, what medication, what dosage, for how long, and what response? Have you been treated with antibiotics? If so, what medications, what dosage, for how long, and what response?

Other Questions Related to Serological Data Have you ever had a "bad blood" test? Were you ever treated for gonorrhea, syphilis, or any sexually transmitted diseases? Is there any history of exposure to risk factors for HIV infection?

There are obviously other questions that could be asked but these questions are of primary importance in interpreting the clinical findings and the results of pertinent blood tests that should be ordered.

Examination

A complete office neuro-ophthalmic examination should be performed on these patients. First, one should look for subtle evidences of aberrant regeneration of the VII nerve that may enable one to confirm a previous bout of peripheral facial nerve palsy. The patient should be instructed to open and close the eyes gently a few times while the examiner looks carefully at the muscles around the chin and mouth to see if there is any subtle intrafacial synkinesis. The pupils should be checked carefully for light-near dissociation. A careful search should be made for any evidence of ocular inflammation; this does not necessarily have to be in a red and painful eye. A careful biomicroscopic examination should be made for a low-grade vitritis with a careful look for anterior and midvitreous cells. One should look carefully for a few small posterior synechiae that might be overlooked if the eye is not inflamed at this time. Particular attention to the fundus periphery with a dilated indirect ophthalmoscopic examination is important to look for pars planitis or evidence of peripheral retinal vasculitis or perivascular sheathing. The optic discs merit close inspection for evidences of perivascular sheathing or high water marks of previous disc swelling as well as any evidence of optic disc pallor. Any signs of iritis, posterior synechiae, vitritis, pars planitis, retinal vasculitis, or optic neuritis should prompt a careful history and a request for a Lyme/treponemal panel.

Laboratory

After a careful history and a complete office neuro-ophthalmologic examination, one must then decide which consultations or laboratory studies to pursue. Only then can one decide, for example, if a magnetic resonance study of the brain is indicated. Although there have been reports of finding white matter lesions in some patients with Lyme borreliosis similar to those seen in patients with multiple sclerosis, it does not mean that every patient with uveitis or pars planitis merits a magnetic resonance scan.

I start by ordering a Lyme/treponemal panel. This test requires the serum from one red-top tube of blood sent to: Microbiology Reference Laboratory (MRL) (10703 Progress Way, Cypress, CA 90630-4714). For a total cost of $90, MRL provides an RPR, FTA-ABS, Lyme IFA IgG and IgM, and a Lyme ELISA. This has been a reliable laboratory in our experience and has been less expensive for this total package than many others we have encountered. It is very important to get all 4 of these tests together at one time, otherwise one could not differentiate the patient whose positive test for Lyme disease was a serological cross-reaction from active or prior syphilitic exposure, and one could not detect the biological false-positive reactor from other autoimmune disease otherwise.

If the patient comes back with a negative Lyme/treponemal panel and the physician still suspects Lyme borreliosis, my practice is to have blood resubmitted to MRL for a serum Western blot and a lymphocyte antigen stimulation test. The patient should come back on a Monday or a Tuesday and have one red-top tube of blood drawn for the Western blot, and two green-top tubes drawn for the lymphocyte stimulation assay. These should be sent by Federal Express at room/ambient temperature (not frozen or refrigerated) to MRL so as to arrive by Wednesday at the latest because the lymphocyte stimulation assay requires living lymphocytes and hence the specimen should not arrive late in the week or on a weekend. The cost for the Western blot test is $45 and the cost for the lymphocyte stimulation assay is $275 when paid to the laboratory. If the patient is billed, the laboratory adds an additional surcharge of approximately 25% for billing. Because the lymphocyte stimulation assay test is so expensive, it should only be ordered on patients who are otherwise seronegative and in whom the physician still has a definite suspicion of the disease.

The polymerase chain reaction test is not available to us through MRL at this time. Preliminary investigation in our department with the urine antigen test has been such that we are not pursuing this test further at this time. When indicated, we send specimens to other laboratories for appropriate confirmation (SmithKline and 3M are excellent laboratories, too). Finally, in special circumstances, we have sent specimens to the Institut Alfred Fournier in Paris to obtain a complete syphilis profile (VDRL, TPHA, TPI, FTA-ABS, FTA-IgM and SPHA-IgM) as well as Lyme IFA and Lyme Western blot tests, for further confirmation. I believe that practitioners will usually be able to resolve the clinical problem by a thorough history, office examination, and use of the Lyme/treponemal panel plus Lyme Western blot tests.

■ Therapeutic Considerations

If a patient is seen with early Lyme borreliosis, oral antibiotics are usually effective. We advise doxycycline (100 mg, 3 times a day) orally for 2 to 3 weeks in such instances. One can also use tetracycline (250 mg, 4 times a day) for 3 to 4 weeks. Erythromycin can be used but has appeared less effective. Ceftin and Suprax have also been used orally. Azithromycin is a new drug under investigation at this time that holds promise of being more effective against *B. burgdorferi.*

Unfortunately, most of the patients seen by ophthalmologists do not present with first-stage Lyme borreliosis but with secondary or tertiary stages of the disease. Furthermore, many have been treated with corticosteroids in the past, which makes eradication of the spirochete more difficult. One can give the patient with iritis or vitritis a course of oral antibiotics (e.g., doxycycline, 100 mg, 3 times a day for 3 weeks), but many patients simply do not respond. It is usually necessary in such cases to administer a course of intravenous antibiotics. Our practice is to have antibiotics administered at home by a visiting nurse via an indwelling heparin-lock venocatheter as a 1-hour infusion each morning. Usually 1 to 2 gm of Rocephin (ceftriaxone; Roche Laboratories, Nutley, NJ) is administered each morning for 30 days. In some cases, if the inflammation is severe and the response to Rocephin seems slow, we have added aqueous penicillin, 3 to 4 million units every 4 hours intravenously via the same regimen. Usually we have relied on Rocephin, however, and the response may be a bit delayed; at times repeat courses of therapy have been necessary. It is not uncommon to have the patient respond to intravenous Rocephin with a definite improvement for 2 to 5 months and then have a recurrence that necessitates retreatment, and again to have the patient respond after that. This reaction is now a controversial aspect of management of Lyme borreliosis and one must try to maintain a balance between creating antibiotic addiction and denying therapy that may really help a distressed individual. Claforan is also used as an intravenous agent for this disease in patients who have not had good responses to Rocephin, but I have too little experience with this drug to comment. I do not hesitate to use topical steroids and cycloplegics in a patient with active uveitis or vitritis along with appropriate antibiotic therapy, but I try to avoid concomitant systemic corticosteroid therapy in patients with suspected Lyme borreliosis whenever possible. Antibiotic therapy in these patients must be continually and carefully evaluated, and the reports by Preac-Mursic and associates [15] of culturing *B. burgdorferi* organisms from patients previously treated with cephtriaxone, doxycycline, and intravenous penicillin must be kept in mind.

■ Controversies in Lyme Borreliosis

Major differences exist at this time in many aspects of this disease. How often does eye involvement occur? At what stages of the disease? What patterns of eye disease are seen? What is "seronegative" Lyme disease? How often does it occur? How is it diagnosed? It is not adequate to exclude this disease by simply saying "the patient has a negative Lyme serology." One must determine which tests were done, at what laboratory, on what date, and what were the exact results. Which cases should be treated with oral versus intravenous antibiotics? Which drugs should be used, in what dosage, and for how long? How extensive a workup should be done? When should repeat courses of therapy be given? What dosage should be used and for how long in such circumstances? Obviously, the answers to these questions will require careful study of the patients with long range follow-up, and the greatest need at this time is not only for an appropriate animal model to study ocular and neurological involvement with Lyme borreliosis, but also to develop a satisfactory and higher yielding method to culture the organism.

■ Thoughts for the Future

The author wrote in 1969 [22] concerning late seronegative syphilis: "The most important point that must now be applied to the management of late syphilis is that there is no necessary correlation between the clinical manifestations of the disease and the serological findings in some cases." This statement is true and applies regardless of the type of serological test used, including the TPI and FTA-ABS tests. Dr Arnold Rich, former professor of pathology at Johns Hopkins Hospital, spent many years studying tuberculosis and concluded in his book *The Pathogenesis of Tuberculosis* [24] that allergy and immunity are different processes. Thus, he found patients dying of tuberculosis who had negative skin tests and others with violent cutaneous reactions were enjoying excellent health. "It is imperative that this concept be transferred from one chronic granulomatous disease (tuberculosis) where the principle is accepted without question, to another chronic granulomatous disease (syphilis) where acceptance of the idea has been slow. The diagnosis of ocular and neurosyphilis and other forms of late syphilis is a *clinical* one and can usually be made with reasonable assurance, no matter what laboratory findings are observed. Another major point is that virulent *Treponema pallidum* organisms are frequently found in aqueous humor, cerebrospinal fluid, and in other tissue sites in the absence of any inflammatory reaction whatever. The Dattner-Thomas hypothesis, that without activity of cerebrospinal fluid (cell count, total protein, colloidal gold curve, or reagin test) there can be no activity of neurosyphilis, has done much to impede recognition of the great problem and prevalence of late syphilis in this country." These comments, which provoked extreme controversy 20 years ago when many considered syphilis as becoming extinct, are not thought to be so heretical now when the incidence of congenital syphilis has gone from only 57 cases in New York City in 1986 to well over 1,000 cases in 1989 [25].

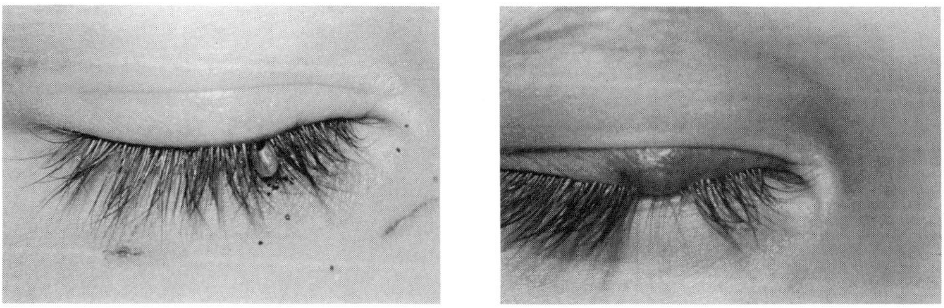

A B

Figure 9 *(A) Tick attached to child's eyelid. (B) Appearance of lid 28 days after removal of tick shows erythema migrans lesion. (Reprinted with permission from Damrow et al [26].)*

If this reasoning holds for syphilis, one suspects that exactly the same situation may prevail with *B. burgdorferi*. This ambiguity will be the challenge confronting neuro-ophthalmological investigators of this disease in the 1990s. Even more basic questions (e.g., controlling the deer population in New England) will have to be faced, but sooner or later, truth must prevail. Finally, one cannot note a more dramatic case of ocular Lyme borreliosis than reported by Damrow and colleagues [26] (Fig 9).

Grateful acknowledgment is given to Dr W. W. Culbertson, Dr Harry Flynn, Dr Kirk Winward, Dr Alan MacDonald, Dr Melvin I. Freeman, A. Paris-Hamelin, Dr Richard Porschen, Dr Wayne Hogrefe, Mrs Barbara French, Mrs Alicia Muniz, Miss Rosa Pelaez, Mr Harry Mayan, Mrs Elvia Ramirez, Mr Omar de Armas, Mrs Ditte Hess, Mrs Linda Duria, Miss Isabel Rams, Mr Ross Jarrett, Mr Antonio Cubillas, and Miss Suzanne Van Meter, for help with this work.

■ References

1. Binder E, Doepfmer R, Hornstein O. Experimentelle ubertragung des erythema chronicum migrans von mensch zu mensch. Hautarzt 1955;6:494–496
2. Sonck CE. Erythema chronicum migrans with multiple lesions. Acta Derm Venereol 1965;45:34–36
3. Burgdorfer W, Barbour AG, Hayes SF, et al. Lyme disease—a tick borne spirochetosis? Science 1982;216:1317–1319
4. Duray PH, Steere AC. Clinical pathologic correlations of Lyme disease by stage. In: Benach JL, Bosler EM, ed. Lyme disease and related disorders. New York: New York Academy of Sciences, 1988:65–79
5. Logigian EL, Kaplan RF, Steere AC. Chronic neurologic manifestations of Lyme disease. N Engl J Med 1990;323:1438–1444
6. Ackermann R, Rehse-Kupper B, Gollmer E, et al. Chronic neurologic manifestations of erythema migrans borreliosis. In: Benach JL, Bosler EM, eds. Lyme disease and related disorders. New York: New York Academy of Sciences, 1988:16–23
7. Steere AC, Duray PH, Kauffmann DJH, et al. Unilateral blindness caused by infection with the Lyme disease spirochete, Borrelia burgdorferi. Ann Intern Med 1985;103:382–384
8. Wu G, Lincoff H, Ellsworth RM, et al. Optic disc edema with Lyme disease. Ann Ophthalmol 1986;18:252–255
9. Winward KE, Smith JL, Culbertson WW, Paris-Hamelin A. Ocular Lyme borreliosis. Am J Ophthalmol 1989;108:651–657
10. Winward KE, Smith JL. Ocular disease in Caribbean patients with serologic evidence of Lyme borreliosis. J Clin Neuro Ophthalmol 1989;9:65–70
11. Duray PH, Johnson RC. The histopathology of experimentally infected hamsters with the Lyme disease spirochete, Borrelia burgdorferi. Proc Soc Exp Biol Med 1986;181:263–269
12. Larsen SA, McGrew BE, Hunter EF, Creighton ET. Syphilis serology and dark-field microscopy. In: Holmes KK, Mardh PA, Sparling PF, Wiesner PJ, eds. Sexually transmitted diseases. New York: McGraw-Hill, 1984:875–888
13. Rawlings JA, Fournier PV, Teltow GJ. Isolation of Borrelia spirochetes from patients in Texas. J Clin Microbiol 1987;25:1148–1150
14. Nadelman RB, Pavia CS, Magnarelli A, et al. Isolation of Borrelia burgdorferi from the blood of seven patients with Lyme disease. Am J Med 1990;88:21–26

15. Preac-Mursic V, Weber K, Pfister HW, et al. Survival of Borrelia burgdorferi in antibiotically treated patients with Lyme borreliosis. Infection 1989;17:355–359
16. Holmes KK. Syphilis. In: Petersdorf RG, Adams RD, Braunwald E, et al, eds. Harrison's principles of internal medicine. New York: McGraw-Hill, 1983:1040
17. Burstain J, Norgard M, Radolf JD. Diagnosis of syphilis by the polymerase chain reaction. JAMA 1990;164:2821 (abstract)
18. Hunter EF, Russell H, Farshy CE, et al. Evaluation of sera from patients with Lyme disease in the fluorescent treponemal antibody-absorption test for syphilis. Sex Transm Dis 1986;12:232–236
19. Harner RE, Smith JL, Israel CW. The FTA-ABS test in late syphilis; review of 1985 cases. JAMA 1968;203:545–548
20. Smith JL, Parsons TM, Paris-Hamelin A, et al. The prevalence of Lyme disease in a nonendemic area. A comparative serologic study in a south Florida eye clinic population. J Clin Neuro Ophthalmol 1989;9:148–155
21. Smith JL, Crumpton BC, Hummer J. The Bascom Palmer Eye Institute Lyme/Syphilis survey. J Clin Neuro Ophthalmol 1990;10:255–260
22. Smith JL. Spirochetes in late seronegative syphilis, penicillin notwithstanding. Springfield, IL: Charles Thomas, 1969
23. Dattwyler RJ, Volkman DJ, Luft BJ, et al. Seronegative Lyme disease. Dissociation of specific T- and B-lymphocyte responses to Borrelia burgdorferi. N Engl J Med 1988;319:1441–1446
24. Rich A. The pathogenesis of tuberculosis. Springfield, IL: Thomas, 1952
25. Dorfman DH, Glaser JH. Congenital syphilis presenting in infants after the newborn period. N Engl J Med 1990;323:1299–1302
26. Damrow T, Freedman H, Lane RS, et al. Is Ixodes (Ixodiopsis) angustus a vector of Lyme disease in Washington State? J West Med 1989;150:580–582

Carotid Endarterectomy and Its Alternatives in Managing Amaurosis Fugax

Jonathan D. Trobe, M.D.

■ What is Carotid Endarterectomy?

The surgical excision of atheroma at the cervical carotid artery bifurcation, called "carotid endarterectomy" (CE), is an accepted treatment of amaurosis fugax and other carotid-distribution transient ischemic attacks. Introduced in 1954 [1], CE grew rapidly in popularity, especially in the United States, where 15,000 procedures were performed in 1971 and 103,000 in 1985, at an estimated cost of $1.2 billion dollars [2]. Other countries have not been as enthusiastic. Only 5% as many CEs were performed in 1980 in the United Kingdom [3]. Even within the United States, one study [4] found a fourfold regional variation in the frequency of CE.

The principal indications for CE have been cerebral and retinal transient ischemic attacks (TIAs) and strokes (50%), and asymptomatic cervical carotid stenosis (50%). A plethora of reports from uncontrolled studies—usually single surgeon or single institution series—have attested to its efficacy in reducing the risk of stroke. There have been only two randomized studies—both flawed. One was completed in the United States in the late 1960s [5], and it reported mild long-term benefit from CE only if the relatively high perioperative casualties (11.5%) were excluded. Its conclusions have been largely ignored because of methodological criticisms. The other randomized study was aborted in 1983 in the United Kingdom because of a 40% stroke/death rate among the first 20 patients to receive CE [6]. As they bowed out, the investigators summed up the problem: "even with the best possible surgical and angiographic technique, there will always be some hazard associated with an operation performed on patients with degenerative vascular disease. With these points in mind, it is clear that convincing benefit from operation will be hard to demonstrate."

More disturbing reports of high morbidity and mortality from CE have appeared in the past decade [7, 8]. A population-based sample of 1,390 cases from three United States sites in 1981 found an aggregate stroke/death rate of 9.8% [9]. At that complication rate, calculations showed that CE provides no improvement on the untreated risk of stroke [10].

No wonder, then, that doubt has begun to gather volume. A 1987 *British Medical Journal* editorialist urged that for asymptomatic carotid stenosis, "spare the knife!" [11]. The American Academy of Neurology's Therapeutics and Technology Assessment Subcommittee [12] and the Stroke Council of the American Heart Association [13] agreed in 1989 that surgeons should not perform CEs unless they could show a perioperative (within 30 days of surgery) stroke/death rate of less than 5% in patients with TIAs.

There has been mounting scrutiny of the indications for CE. A panel of experts determined that only 35% of 1,302 CEs performed in three sites in the United States in 1981 were "appropriate" [9]. Applying the same standards, 55% of 107 CEs performed in five Veterans Administration hospitals in 1981 were judged "appropriate" [14]. The impact of these findings has been palpable. Between 1985 and 1986, the number of CEs performed nationwide dropped from 103,000 to 81,000 [15].

Where does this controversy leave ophthalmologists trying to manage patients with amaurosis fugax? In a serious quandary. The natural (untreated) risk of hemispheric stroke after an attack of transient monocular blindness (TMB) is probably lower than that after a hemispheric TIA. Yet the risk of death (usually from myocardial infarction) is equal to that after a hemispheric TIA. One-third of patients will die within five years [16], and CE has never been shown to increase that life span. Thus, CE must work its stroke-reducing magic within a relatively narrow "window of opportunity." To offer benefit in patients who have TMB as their only manifestation of brain ischemia, CE surgeons must theoretically provide a serious complication rate even lower than the 5% suggested for hemispheric TIAs.

In truth, no one really knows if CE actually reduces the risk of stroke after TMB or any TIA. Two large randomized trials (one in North America, the other in Europe) are underway and should have some answers by 1993. The North American Symptomatic Carotid Endarterectomy Trial (NASCET) released an interim preliminary report on February 25, 1991, announcing that CE appears to reduce the risk of stroke by 17% within 18 months in patients with stenosis greater than 70% who have had prior carotid artery–distribution minor stroke or TIAs. The perioperative (30-day) morbidity and mortality was only 2% among 300 CE patients. The 295 patients treated with antiplatelet agents had a 3% stroke morbidity and mortality rate within 30 days.

■ Where Did Carotid Endarterectomy Come From?

In 1952, in a report of a series of patients with episodes of transient contralateral hemiplegia and TMB, Fisher [17] argued that intermittent carotid occlusion was not the causative mechanism because (1) the two symptoms never seemed to occur together, and (2) surgical ligation of the cervical carotid rarely gave rise to TMB. Drawing on the previous fundus observations of others who had uniformly noted "retinal pallor associated with bloodless, thread-like arteries" [17], Fisher suggested that vasospasm close to the eye was the explanation for TMB. Seven years later, as he watched "white segments" traverse the fundus within retinal arterioles during episodes of TMB, he changed his mind. He now considered embolism the cause, and the cervical carotid the likely source [18]. Over the next few years, others [19, 20] would draw the same conclusions.

Soon there was a credible link between TMB, hemispheric TIA, and cervical carotid atheroma. David and associates [21] reported that the intraretinal "bright plaques" consisted pathologically of cholesterol esters identical to those recovered from the carotid lesion. Similar emboli were found in an occluded middle cerebral artery. McBrien and colleagues [22] found white particles in retinal arterioles following CE that proved histologically to consist of platelet aggregates. Had they reached their destination from the cervical carotid atheroma? Gunning and co-workers [23] provided circumstantial evidence by finding that patients with recent TMB had a loose network of fibrin on their carotid plaques during CE, whereas those with remote TMB had no such friable surface.

It soon became apparent that atherostenotic lesions and ulcerated plaques were present in the extracranial carotid artery in a majority of older adults with TMB and other TIAs. Fortuitously, the extracranial atheromas were far more common (at least in Caucasians) in the surgically accessible extracranial portion than the intracranial portion of the carotid artery. It was not unusual to find near obliteration of the lumen at the cervical carotid bifurcation with apparently normal distal circuits. Most anterior (carotid) circulation TIAs and strokes, including those involving the eye, were ascribed to carotid occlusion or embolism [24]. Either way, lesion excision would theoretically be preventative. The rationale for CE was born.

The rationale provided a wide latitude. Any irregularity in the luminal surface might be the nidus for an embolus. Vertebrobasilar TIAs in the presence of carotid stenosis would be reduced by CE because it provided more blood flow to the posterior circulation through the arterial circle of Willis. As it became clear that asymptomatic carotid stenosis was itself a marker for future stroke, that too became an indication for CE. Within the past decade, asymptomatic patients have constituted 25 to 50% of those undergoing CE; among the symptomatic patients, vertebrobasilar TIAs have made up approximately 10%, and TMB patients approximately 10 to 15%. Within this theoretical backdrop, however, some weak spots began to appear.

Angiographically Normal Cervical Carotids

A sizeable proportion of elderly patients with TIAs have normal angiograms. Among others, Adams and associates [25] reported that only one-third of 59 older adult patients with TMB had significant carotid atheromas and one-third had completely normal angiograms.

Failure of Bypass Procedure

In 1985, the results of a massive collaborative study [26] showed that anastomosing the superficial temporal artery to the middle cerebral artery (extracranial–intracranial bypass) to circumvent an occluded carotid does not reduce the risk of stroke. This outcome dealt a crushing blow to the notion that CE worked by providing more blood to the brain, at least in chronic cervical occlusive disease. That left only two possibilities: CE reduces the risk of acute carotid occlusion or embolism.

The Stereotypic Nature of TMB

Ever since Fisher's 1952 report [17], observers have had difficulty explaining how cervical carotid emboli could account for the stereotyped and isolated nature of TMB, which often has the same altitudinal pattern in attack after attack. Notwithstanding that experiments have shown that artificial emboli tend to travel up the same circuits [27], vasoocclusive factors closer to the eye are a more logical explanation of TMB, as Fisher [17] had originally suggested.

Other Possible Mechanisms

The heart has been recognized as a possible source of brain emboli. Unfortunately, neither the patient's description of visual loss nor any other clinical indicator is reliable in differentiating a carotid from a cardiac source of emboli [28]. In fact, it is even difficult to distinguish migraine from thromboembolism as a cause of TMB [29]. "Hypercoagulable states" have been described in which thrombi seem to form without a mural nidus [30, 31].

Regardless of the rationale, the advisability of CE for patients with TMB and other TIAs must be judged on results: Does it or does it not reduce future stroke and at what cost?

■ What are the Results of Carotid Endarterectomy?

The two most reliable, but uncontrolled, follow-up studies of CE have shown a 0.9% [32] and 1.7% [33] yearly stroke rate. These rates are a spectacular improvement over the expected annual rate of 6% in surgically untreated hemispheric TIA patients followed in Rochester, Minnesota [34], and in aspirin-treated subjects [35, 36]. But is it a major improvement over the natural risk of stroke in patients with TMB only?

The data on the untreated course of TMB patients are sketchy. The landmark 1968 study by Marshall and Meadows [37] showed a hemispheric stroke rate of 1.2% per year and a retinal stroke rate of 2.5% per year. The principal drawback was that fewer than one-third of patients had cerebral angiography. Even so, subsequent studies with more comprehensive angiography and follow-up are showing similar stroke rates after TMB. A 1985 study at Duke University [38] followed 35 patients with TMB and angiographically verified ipsilateral carotid stenosis for an average of seven years with an estimated yearly stroke rate of 2%. By comparison, patients with hemispheric TIA had twice the annual stroke rate (4%). Poole and Ross-Russell [39] found nearly identical results: a yearly stroke rate of 2.2% in 110 patients followed for six years.

If the stroke rate after TMB appears to be approximately 2% per year, it is apparently higher for patients with retinal emboli or stroke—perhaps equal to the 4 to 6% per year stroke rate for patients with hemispheric TIA [40–42].

How may we explain the discrepancy between the low stroke rate after TMB and the relatively higher stroke rate after retinal emboli, infarct, and hemispheric TIA? There are two theories. (1) TMB requires a "smaller amount" of ischemia than does hemispheric TIA. Unlike other parts of the cerebrum, the anterior visual pathway has no anatomical reduplication. Moreover, temporary visual loss is more likely to draw the patient's attention than temporary numbness or weakness of the limbs. (2) TMB is less commonly a manifestation of atherosclerotic cerebrovascular disease than is hemispheric TIA. Migraine, for example, causes visual loss more than any other neurological deficit. If the relatively low stroke risk of TMB is real, then a postoperative stroke risk of 1 to 2% per year provided by CE will not be much of an improvement over the natural course. Even for patients with retinal emboli/infarct, CE may not be worthwhile unless the perioperative stroke/death rate is below 3%.

■ What are the Hazards of Carotid Endarterectomy?

There are two serious immediate complications from CE: nonfatal but disabling stroke and fatal myocardial infarction. These two events occur with a frequency that varies from 2 to 24% among published reports [43]. Stroke occurs approximately three times as often as myocardial infarction. The lowest complication rates tend to come from single surgeon or single institution series, such as one from the University of Alabama reviewing 142 consecutive CEs performed from 1979 to 1985 with an overall serious complication rate of 2.1% [44]. Much higher complication rates come from community studies or external reviews: (1) five Veterans Administration hospitals, 107 procedures, 1981, 5.6% [14]; (2) Medicare claims from 139 New England hospitals, 2,089 procedures, 1984 to 1985, 7.5% [45]; (3) Medicare claims from three selected United States sites, 1,302 procedures, 1981, 9.8% [9]; (4) chart review from 16 Cincinnati community hospitals, 431 procedures, 1980, 11.4% [46]; and (5) chart review by the same authors from the same 16 Cincinnati hospitals, 750 procedures, 1983 to 1984, 7.4% [47]. Why are there such outcome discrepancies between the "choice series" and the "outside reviews?" One possible explanation came from a 1980 study by two neurologists who did a "page-by-page" review of the medical records of 431 CEs performed in 16 Cincinnati community hospitals. Only 15 of the 37 perioperative strokes were recorded in the hospital discharge summaries [46].

Are there any patient or surgeon characteristics that correlate with especially bad outcomes? With regard to patients, studies generally show that complications are more frequent if patients have angiographic, medical, or neurological risk factors. Sundt and colleagues [48], from the Mayo Clinic, defined four incremental risk groups.

Grade I. No medical, neurological, or angiographic risk factors with unilateral or bilateral carotid stenosis.

Grade II. No medical or neurological risk factors, but one or more of the following angiographic risk factors: coexisting siphon stenosis, extensive carotid plaque with distal extension to level of second cervical vertebra, contralateral carotid occlusion, or evidence of a soft thrombus within the carotid lesion.

Grade III. No neurological risk factors, but one or more of the following medical risk factors: angina pectoris, myocardial infarction within six months, blood pressure greater than 180/110, chronic obstructive pulmonary disease, severe obesity, or age greater than 70 years. Angiographic risk factors may or may not be present.

Grade IV. One or more of the following neurological risk factors: progressing neurological deficit, fixed deficit less than 24 hours old, or multiple deficits owing to multiple strokes. Medical or angiographic risk factors may or may not be present.

With regard to the characteristics of surgeons or the operative technique, no reproducible findings have emerged. Oddly, the surgeon's specialty and case volume have not influenced the results. A reasonable conclusion is that there is an irreducible minimum complication rate imposed by the fact that most candidates for CE have widespread atherosclerosis. In the best of hands, they are prone to perioperative stroke and myocardial infarction.

■ What is the Role of Carotid Endarterectomy?

Given these sobering facts, most observers have agreed that it is time for a serious reappraisal of CE. As the results of the randomized trials comparing CE to aspirin are eagerly awaited, some useful guidelines have emerged.

In a respected decision-analysis, Matchar and Pauker [49] decided that a 5% major complication rate for CE was probably the lowest one could reasonably promise the patient, based on published reports. Even at that complication rate, they recommended that no CE be performed if the untreated stroke risk is less than 3%. Until better information is available, we must assume that patients with TMB fall within that domain. Matchar and Pauker [49] also concluded that even if the untreated risk of stroke is between 3 and 5% per year, "surgery can be expected to provide a benefit of at most three months of quality life." For patients with retinal emboli and infarct, the untreated yearly stroke risk probably falls within that 3 to 5% range. Considering that no large study has ever analyzed the post-CE stroke rate in patients with retinal emboli or infarct who have not had recent TIAs, one cannot recommend CE enthusiastically for this group either. A reasonable approach is to consider CE only if the patient falls within Mayo Clinic Grade I or II risk groups and the surgeon has a "track record" of an extremely low complication rate (<3%). CE should be performed only if carotid stenosis is greater than 70% (hemodynamically significant) and there are no Mayo Clinic angiographic risk factors.

There are three other manifestations of visual system ischemia about which ophthalmologists must make a decision regarding CE.

Ischemic Optic Neuropathy

The long-term clinical course of patients with nonarteritic anterior ischemic optic neuropathy (NAION) is not well documented. In one follow-up study of 205 patients with NAION [50], there was a slightly greater incidence of stroke and myocardial infarction than expected, but no greater mortality.

A retrospective study of 71 patients with NAION showed a two- to threefold higher myocardial and cerebral infarction mortality than expected [51]. The pathogenesis of NAION, however, is believed to be nonembolic occlusion of small ciliary arterioles within the optic nervehead. Although carotid stenosis is a common finding, it should be managed as if the patient were asymptomatic. The advisability of CE in patients with asymptomatic carotid stenosis is controversial and is the subject of two current randomized trials with anticipated completion dates in 1993 [12].

Visual Loss from Cortical Ischemia

Homonymous or other binocular visual loss generally results from ischemia of striate cortex mediated by vertebrobasilar or cardiac thromboembolism. Given the failure of extracranial-intracranial bypass, the concept of opening up the "front door" (carotid system) when the "back door" (vertebrobasilar system) is tight has no foundation. There is no role for CE in this situation.

Ocular Ischemic Syndrome (OIS)

Chronic ischemia to the globe may be manifested in the retina (i.e., venous dilatation and hemorrhage, capillary nonperfusion, prolonged retinal vascular transit time, cotton wool spots, neovascularization) and anterior segment (i.e., anterior chamber flare, cataract, hypotony, rubeosis iridis) [52, 53]. This condition is closely associated with severe ipsilateral carotid stenosis; on the other hand, it is rare even in patients with complete carotid occlusion [54]. Because the same findings may be found in ophthalmic artery obstruction [55], chances are that OIS is caused by vascular insufficiency closer to the eye than the cervical carotid artery. Isolated reports describe resolution of signs of ocular ischemia after CE [56] and extracranial–intracranial bypass [57]. These Mayo-Clinic "cry-in-the-wilderness" descriptions, however, have not been duplicated, probably because atherosclerotic disease is so advanced in these patients that surgical morbidity is high. Panretinal photocoagulation (PRP) has been effective in reversing rubeosis iridis after ischemic central retinal vein occlusion [58], a condition that is related to OIS. Limited experience with PRP in the OIS, however, has been discouraging [53].

■ Are There Alternatives to Carotid Endarterectomy?

The medical management of TMB and other TIAs consists of reducing the modifiable arteriosclerotic risk factors and prescribing platelet antiaggregants. This approach presumes that TMB is caused by factors related to arteriosclerosis, a reasonable presumption in adults over the age of 40 in whom migraine and other pertinent nonarteriosclerotic conditions have been excluded.

Among modifiable risk factors for stroke, hypertension is dominant. Men with blood pressures greater than 160/95 have a fivefold greater likelihood of stroke than men with blood pressures less than 140/90 [59]. Systolic hypertension alone, a common finding among the elderly, is as ominous a risk factor for stroke as diastolic hypertension. Obesity, cigarette smoking, and probably alcoholism are separate and important risk factors [59]. The relationship of sedentary life-style and blood lipids (including cholesterol) to stroke is not as clear as it is to coronary artery disease [59]. The relationship between oral contraceptives and TMB, TIA, and stroke is controversial. Although an increased risk has been shown, it is principally in women over 35 years of age who smoke and have hypertension. Most of the data apply to the higher doses of estrogen that are no longer prescribed [60].

Among the platelet antiaggregants, aspirin has proved its worth as a stroke risk reducer, but only modestly. An impressive analysis of all aspirin-in-stroke–prevention trials has shown that aspirin reduces stroke by 14% [61]. (Compare this figure to the 50% or better stroke risk reduction by CE suggested by uncontrolled studies.) Doses of 325 mg per day (one adult tablet) have been found to be as effective as higher doses and less likely to cause bleeding and gastrotoxicity [61].

Ticlopidine hydrochloride, a new platelet antiaggregant that affects cell membranes rather than prostaglandins, was shown to be as effective as aspirin in two large randomized trials [62, 63]. Nausea, diarrhea, leukopenia, and skin rash occurring in 1 to 5% of patients may limit its acceptance. The two other platelet antiaggregants, sulfinpyrazone (Anturane R) and dipyridamole (Persantine R) [64] have no place in the prevention of stroke.

Heparin [65] and warfarin [66] anticoagulants have never been shown to prevent stroke in controlled trials. Even so, they are sometimes used in desperation. Conventional doses of warfarin that prolong the prothrombin time to twice normal are associated with a dangerously high rate of bleeding; lower doses, aimed at prolonging the prothrombin time to 1.25 times normal, may be as effective and much less hazardous [67].

■ What Should Ophthalmologists Do?

Confronted with a patient who has transient visual loss, ophthalmologists' first task is to decide if the deficit derives from the anterior (globe or optic nerve) or posterior (retrochiasmal) visual pathway. If the visual loss is binocular, CE is never a consideration. If the visual loss is monocular (TMB), ophthalmologists must first rule out a nonatherosclerotic cause, such as migraine, papilledema, or sickle cell retinopathy. If these are negative, one should next rule out a cardiac source of embolism such as valvular disease or arrhythmia. If atherosclerotic risk factors, symptoms, or signs are present, cervical carotid thromboembolism must also be considered. At this point, however, management becomes controversial. Current evidence of the risks and benefits of CE do not support its use for patients with any ocular manifestations of acute ischemia [68] (Figure). In chronic ocular ischemia (OIS), reported studies of CE are too few to judge its value. The ongoing randomized trials may show that CE has a role in some of these ocular conditions. Until then, ophthalmologists should be wary of "feeding the stream" that leads to CE. Only if Mayo Grade I to II patients with unequivocal, recent symptoms can be matched with surgeons with demonstrably low perioperative stroke/death rates should CE

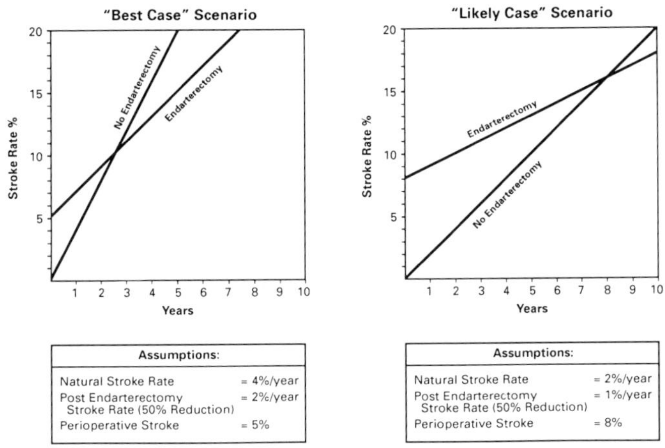

Comparison of the chance of stroke with and without carotid endarterectomy using two sets of assumptions. In the "best case" scenario (left), *where a relatively high natural stroke rate and low perioperative stroke rate are used, the risk of stroke with endarterectomy is higher for only the first 3 years. In the "likely case" scenario* (right), *where a more realistic natural stroke rate and perioperative stroke rate are used, the risk of stroke with endarterectomy is higher for 8 years after the procedure.*

even be considered. Duplex carotid ultrasound is a cost-effective method of screening such patients for angiography [69].

For most patients with visual system ischemia, attention should center on the broader issues of medical management, namely the manipulation of risk factors. Leaf and Ryan [70] wrote that "such a shift in perceptions will require substantial cultural changes by both physicians and the public. Members of the public will need to accept more responsibility for their own health . . . they will need to be disabused of the fantasy that . . . medicine will make available a pill or operation to erase the adverse health effects of a lifetime of self-abuse." They were referring to coronary artery disease, but the message applies equally to amaurosis fugax, cerebrovascular disease, and CE.

■ References

1. Eastcott HHG, Pickering GW, Rob CG. Reconstruction of internal carotid artery in a patient with intermittent attacks of hemiplegia. Lancet 1954;2:994–996
2. Dyken ML, Pokras R. The performance of endarterectomy for disease of the extracranial arteries of the head. Stroke 1984;15:948–950
3. Warlow C, Whisnant JP, Dyken ML. Carotid endarterectomy. In: Plum F, Pulsinelli W, eds. Cerebrovascular diseases. New York: Raven, 1985:43–48
4. Chassin MR, Brook RH, Park RE, et al. Variations in the use of medical and surgical services by the Medicare population. N Engl J Med 1986;314:285–290
5. Fields WS, Maslenikov V, Meyer JS, et al. Joint study of extracranial arterial occlusion. V. Progress report of prognosis following surgery or nonsurgical treatment

for transient cerebral ischemic attacks and cervical carotid artery lesions. JAMA 1970;211:1993–2003

6. Shaw DA, Venable GS, Cartlidge NEF, et al. Carotid endarterectomy in patients with transient cerebral ischemia. J Neurol Sci 1984;64:45–53
7. Warlow C. Carotid endarterectomy: does it work? Stroke 1984;15:1068–1075
8. Brott TG, Labutta RJ, Kempczinski RF. Changing patterns in the practice of carotid endarterectomy in a large metropolitan area. JAMA 1986;255:2609–2612
9. Winslow CM, Solomon DH, Chassin MR, et al. The appropriateness of carotid endarterectomy. N Engl J Med 1988;318:721–727
10. Committee on Health Care Issues, American Neurological Association. Does carotid endarterectomy decrease stroke and death in patients with transient ischemic attacks? Ann Neurol 1987;22:72–76
11. Sandercock P. Asymptomatic carotid stenosis: spare the knife. Br Med J 1987;294:1368
12. American Academy of Neurology Therapeutics and Technology Assessment Committee. Interim assessment: carotid endarterectomy. Neurology 1990;40:682–683
13. Beebe HG, Clagett P, DeWeese JA, et al. Assessing risk associated with carotid endarterectomy. A statement for health professionals by an ad hoc committee on carotid surgery standards of the Stroke Council, American Heart Association. Stroke 1989;20:314–315
14. Merrick NJ, Brook RH, Fink A, et al. Use of carotid endarterectomy in five California Veterans Administration medical centers. JAMA 1986;256:2531–2535
15. Pokras R, Dyken ML. Dramatic changes in the performance of endarterectomy for diseases of the extracranial arteries of the head. Stroke 1988;19:1289–1290
16. Heyman A, Wilkinson WE, Hurwitz BJ, et al. Risk of ischemic heart disease in patients with TIA. Neurology 1984;34:626–630
17. Fisher CM. Transient monocular blindness associated with hemiplegia. Arch Ophthalmol 1952;47:167–203
18. Fisher CM. Observations of the fundus oculi in transient monocular blindness. Neurology 1959;9:337–347
19. Ross-Russell RW. Observations on the retinal vessels in monocular blindness. Lancet 1961;2:1422–1425
20. Hollenhorst RW. Significance of bright plaques in the retinal arterioles. JAMA 1961;178:23–29
21. David NJ, Klintworth GK, Friedberg SJ, et al. Fatal atheromatous cerebral embolism associated with bright plaques in retinal arterioles. Report of a case. Neurology 1963;13:708–713
22. McBrien DJ, Bradley RD, Ashton N. The nature of retinal emboli in stenosis of the internal carotid artery. Lancet 1963;1:697–710
23. Gunning AJ, Pickering GW, Robb-Smith AHT, et al. Mural thrombosis of the internal carotid artery and subsequent embolism. Q J Med 1964;33:155–164
24. Mohr JP, Pessin MS. Extracranial carotid artery disease. In: Barnett HJM, Stein BM, Mohr JP, Yatsu FM, eds. Stroke. Pathophysiology, diagnosis, and management. New York: Churchill Livingstone, 1986:304–313
25. Adams HP, Putman SF, Corbett JJ, et al. Amaurosis fugax: the results of arteriography in 59 patients. Stroke 1983;14:742–744
26. The EC/IC Bypass Study Group. Failure of extracranial–intracranial arterial bypass to reduce the risk of ischemic stroke: results of an international randomized trial. N Engl J Med 1985;313:1191–1200
27. Whisnant JP. Multiple particles injected may all go to the same cerebral artery branch. Stroke 1982;13:720–724
28. Bogousslavsky J, Hachinski V, Boughner D, et al. Clinical predictors of cardiac and arterial lesions in carotid transient ischemic attacks. Arch Neurol 1986;43:229–233

29. Goodwin JA, Gorelick PB, Helgason CM. Symptoms of amaurosis fugax in atherosclerotic carotid artery disease. Neurology 1987;37:829–832
30. Schafer AI. The hypercoagulable states. Ann Intern Med 1985;102:814–828
31. Asherson RA, Khamashta MA, Gil A, et al. Cerebrovascular disease and antiphospholipid antibodies in systemic lupus erythematosus, lupus-like disease, and the primary antiphospholipid syndrome. Am J Med 1989;86:391–399
32. Sundt TM, Whisnant JP, Houser OW, et al. Prospective study of the effectiveness and durability of carotid endarterectomy. Mayo Clin Proc 1990;65:625–635
33. Turner DA, Tracy J, Haines SJ. Risk of late stroke and survival following carotid endarterectomy procedures for symptomatic patients. J Neurosurg 1990;73:193–200
34. Matsumoto N, Whisnant JP, Kurland LT, et al. Natural history of stroke in Rochester, Minnesota, 1955 through 1969: an extension of a previous study, 1945 through 1954. Stroke 1973;4:20–29
35. Canadian Cooperative Study Group. A randomized trial of aspirin and sulfinpyrazone in threatened stroke. N Engl J Med 1978;299:53–59
36. Fields WS, Lemak NA, Frankowski RF, et al. Controlled trial of aspirin in cerebral ischemia. Stroke 1977;8:301–316
37. Marshall J, Meadows S. The natural history of amaurosis fugax. Brain 1968;91:419–434
38. Hurwitz BJ, Heyman A, Wilkinson WE, et al. Comparison of amaurosis fugax and transient cerebral ischemia: a prospective clinical and arteriographic study. Ann Neurol 1985;18:698–704
39. Poole C, Ross-Russell R. Mortality and stroke after amaurosis fugax. J Neurol Neurosurg Psychiatry 1985;48:902–905
40. Howard RS, Ross-Russell RW. Prognosis of patients with retinal embolism. J Neurol Neurosurg Psychiatry 1987;50:1142–1147
41. Savino PJ, Glaser JS, Cassady J. Retinal stroke: is the patient at risk? Arch Ophthalmol 1982;89:1336–1347
42. Pfaffenbach DD, Hollenhorst RW. Morbidity and survivorship of patients with embolic cholesterol crystals in the ocular fundus. Am J Ophthalmol 1966;61:1159–1165
43. Cebul RD, Whisnant JP. Carotid endarterectomy. Ann Intern Med 1989;111:660–670
44. Zeiger HE, Zampella EJ, Naftel DC, et al. A prospective analysis of 142 carotid endarterectomies for occlusive vascular disease, 1979–1985. J Neurosurg 1987;67:540–544
45. Fisher ES, Malenka DJ, Solomon NA, et al. Risk of carotid endarterectomy in the elderly. Am J Public Health 1989;79:1617–1620
46. Brott T, Thalinger K. The practice of carotid endarterectomy in a large metropolitan area. Stroke 1984;15:950–955
47. Brott TG, Labutta RJ, Kempczinski RF. Changing patterns in the practice of carotid endarterectomy in a large metropolitan area. JAMA 1986;255:2609–2612
48. Sundt TM Jr, Sandok BA, Whisnant JP. Carotid endarterectomy: complications and preoperative assessment of risk. Mayo Clin Proc 1975;50:301–306
49. Matchar DB, Pauker SG. Endarterectomy in carotid artery disease. A decision analysis. JAMA 1987;258:793–798
50. Guyer DR, Miller NR, Auer CL, et al. The risk of cerebrovascular and cardiovascular disease in patients with anterior ischemic optic neuropathy. Arch Ophthalmol 1985;103:1136–1142
51. Sawle GV, James CB, Ross-Russell RW. The natural history of non-arteritic anterior ischaemic optic neuropathy. J Neurol Neurosurg Psychiatry 1990;53:830–833
52. Knox DL. Ischemic ocular inflammation. Am J Ophthalmol 1965;60:995–1002

53. Brown GC, Coscas G, Gutman FA, et al. Ophthalmic manifestations of carotid artery disease. In: Singerman LK, Jampol LM, eds. Retinal and choroidal manifestations of systemic disease. Baltimore: Williams & Wilkins, 1991:128–146
54. Kearns TP, Siebert RG. The ocular aspects of carotid artery surgery. Trans Am Ophthalmol Soc 1978;76:247–265
55. Brown GC, Magargal LF, Simeone FA, et al. Arterial obstruction and ocular neovascularization. Ophthalmology 1982;89:139–146
56. Neupert JR, Brubaker RF, Kearns TP, et al. Rapid resolution of venous stasis retinopathy after carotid endarterectomy. Am J Ophthalmol 1976;81:600–602
57. Kearns TP, Younge BR, Piepgras DG. Resolution of venous stasis retinopathy after carotid artery bypass surgery. Mayo Clin Proc 1980;55:342–346
58. Magargal LE, Brown GC, Augsburger JJ, et al. Efficacy of panretinal photocoagulation in preventing neovascular glaucoma following ischemic central retinal vein obstruction. Ophthalmol 1982;89:780–784
59. Wolf PA, Kannel WB, McGee DL. Prevention of ischemic stroke: risk factors. In: Barnett HJM, Stein BM, Mohr JP, Yatsu FM, eds. Stroke: Pathophysiology, diagnosis, and management. New York: Churchill Livingstone, 1986:967–988
60. Longstreth W, Koepsell T, Yerby M, et al. Risk factors for subarachnoid hemorrhage. Stroke 1985;16:377–385
61. Antiplatelet Trialists' Collaboration. Secondary prevention of vascular disease by prolonged antiplatelet treatment. Br Med J 1988;196:316–320
62. Hass WK, Easton JD, Adams HP, et al. A randomized trial comparing ticlopidine hydrochloride with aspirin for the prevention of stroke in high-risk patients. N Engl J Med 1989;321:501–507
63. Gent M, Blakely JA, Easton JD, et al. The Canadian American Ticlopidine Study (CATS) in thromboembolic stroke. Lancet 1989;1:1215–1220
64. Fitzgerald GA. Dipyridamole. N Engl J Med 1987;316:1247–1256
65. Keith DS, Phillips SJ, Whisnant JP, et al. Heparin therapy for recent transient focal cerebral ischemia. Mayo Clin Proc 1987;62:1101–1106
66. Grotta JC. Current medical and surgical therapy for cerebrovascular disease. N Engl J Med 1987;317:1505–1516
67. Hirsh J, Levine M. Therapeutic range for the control of oral anticoagulant therapy. Arch Neurol 1986;43:1162–1164
68. Trobe JD. Carotid endarterectomy. Who needs it? Ophthalmology 1987;94: 725–730
69. Hankey GJ, Warlow CP. Symptomatic carotid ischaemic events: safest and most cost effective way of selecting patients for angiography, before carotid endarterectomy. Br Med J 1990;300:1485–1491
70. Leaf A, Ryan TJ. Prevention of coronary artery disease. A medical imperative. N Engl J Med 1990;323:1416–1419

Automated Perimetry in Neuro-ophthalmology

Richard P. Mills, M.D.

Testing the visual field occupies a central position in neuro-ophthalmic examinations. The importance accorded such testing is appropriate because of the high frequency of visual pathway involvement in patients with neurological disease. Among the ophthalmic subspecialties, only glaucoma shares with neuro-ophthalmology this emphasis on visual field testing.

As automated threshold perimeters became available, they enjoyed rapid acceptance among physicians specializing in glaucoma who recognized their superiority in detecting the earliest perimetric signs of damage. The enthusiasm of neuro-ophthalmologists for the new technique has been more restrained for a number of reasons.

First, although the vast majority of glaucoma patients can cooperate reasonably well throughout a rather lengthy visual field test, there are a significant number of patients with neurological disease who cannot. Automated perimeters with currently available software do not detect these marginally cooperative patients and automatically change strategy or abbreviate the test, as good perimetrists using manual methods have always done. Consequently, some neuro-ophthalmology patients may perform so poorly during automated perimetry that the entire field testing exercise is viewed as counterproductive.

Second, there are often different expectations of visual field testing in glaucoma and neuro-ophthalmology. In glaucoma, the emphasis is on finding the earliest field changes of the disease or on documenting the smallest increment of change that is significant. Such findings are a sufficient condition to result directly in a change in patient treatment. In neuro-ophthalmology, the emphasis is usually on topical diagnosis, the determination of the site of visual pathway involvement. Only rarely is the visual field information the sole criterion for a treatment decision. In a generic sense, the requirement in neuro-ophthalmology is most often for a good qualitative field, whereas in glaucoma quantitative needs prevail.

Third, patients with neuro-ophthalmic disease usually require different visual field interpretation strategies than patients with glaucoma. In patients with glaucoma, careful attention to the nasal horizontal meridian is necessary to detect subtle steps, whereas in neuro-ophthalmology, the vertical meridian is the more important factor to detect chiasmal and retrochiasmal lesions. In the software of the Humphrey (Allergan–Humphrey, San Leandro, CA) and the Octopus (Interzeag AG, Schlieren, Switzerland) automated perimeters, statistical analysis packages for the threshold visual field data are designed to detect glaucomatous visual field defects and to follow them over time. No comparable commercial software packages are available for neuro-ophthalmic applications.

Although these three objections of automated perimetry in neuro-ophthalmology have a measure of validity, they are not sufficient to discourage comprehensive ophthalmologists from harnessing the automated perimeter in the service of patients with neuro-ophthalmic disease. In fact, once an ophthalmologist is armed with understanding of the strengths and weaknesses of automated field testing and the confidence that he or she can interpret the results properly, automated testing offers many benefits over conventional manual testing methods.

Even the objections listed earlier seem less objectionable. It turns out that most patients with suspected neuro-ophthalmic disease have no associated neurological disease that prevents optimal cooperation during perimetry; in fact, many such patients are young and perform quite well for testing. Patients with pseudotumor cerebri and papilledema or Graves' disease and threatened optic nerve decompensation need sensitive quantitative testing. Finally, a different interpretation strategy for evaluating an automated field chart is all that is required to optimize the diagnostic information obtained.

This chapter will cover first some basic principles of perimetry as they apply to testing neuro-ophthalmology patients. Then, choice of test will be discussed. Finally, an interpretive strategy will be presented, illustrated with examples of Humphrey automated fields from patients with disease at different levels of the afferent visual system.

■ Types of Perimetry

Before the introduction of automated perimetry, clinical visual field testing used a kinetic method in which the stimulus was moved from a nonseeing area of the visual field toward the seeing area. The point at which patients first see the stimulus was marked. After testing many points with the same stimulus, the points could be connected by a line called an isopter. One or many isopters could be drawn to map the field of vision, and ophthalmologists felt comfortable interpreting the resulting charts from the Goldmann perimeter or tangent screen. Modifications of the kinetic testing method featuring spot checking with static stimuli within the central field, such as the Armaly-Drance strategy, increased sensitivity in detecting glaucoma and other diseases.

The kinetic method has some disadvantages that were not commonly recognized until an alternative testing method was available. For example, depressions in visual field sensitivity that do not extend peripherally to the outer isopter are easy to miss unless perimetrists are fortunate enough to begin testing within the scotoma. In most circumstances, visual sensitivity drops off gradually with distance from the center, but in those cases without much drop-off in sensitivity, isopters are difficult to plot accurately. Additionally, moving stimuli are easier to detect within defective areas of the field than those that are standing still. Most important, because total automation of the kinetic method has not been achievable, kinetic perimetry requires highly trained, skilled perimetrists to achieve valid results, a situation that is not common in many ophthalmology offices.

Static perimetry uses stimuli that do not move but are illuminated for short durations, usually under 0.5 second. If each point is tested with an appropriate range of stimulus strengths, an estimate can be made of the threshold, which is the minimum strength needed for the stimulus to be seen at least half the time. An array of points strategically located throughout the visual field at which threshold has been estimated constitutes a static threshold test. This quantitative method of testing is quite time-consuming but is the most sensitive for detecting early damage within the central visual field.

If static stimuli are presented just brighter than the expected threshold at many points in the field, a chart can be constructed that records points seen with one symbol and points missed with another. Because multiple presentations at each point are not used, this suprathreshold static testing method is quite fast but produces only qualitative information. It is therefore limited to screening for defects, not for following established ones over time. The usefulness of the method is enhanced by advance knowledge of the expected thresholds across a patient's visual field, either from previous threshold test results or from a few threshold values obtained at the beginning of the threshold-related suprathreshold static test.

Currently available automated perimeters perform static threshold testing. The most common pattern employed for such testing has points separated by 6 degrees of visual angle in a regular array within the central 30 degrees (e.g., Octopus 38, Humphrey 30-2). Although software is available for static threshold testing in the peripheral field, the variability of response is quite large in the periphery, and the incremental information may not be worth the additional time investment.

The Humphrey automated perimeter has optional kinetic test software available. As currently constituted, it tests only peripheral isopters and requires involvement by technicians to perform more than basic screening.

■ Visual Field Tasks in Neuro-ophthalmology

In general, there are three levels of visual field testing: screening for abnormality, screening for diagnosis, and quantitation. In screening for abnormality, the object is to discover if a visual field is normal. Such screening is appropriate in patients with a very low probability of disease, when the decreased sensitivity is an acceptable trade-off for the short duration of the test. In screening for diagnosis, a more involved test is administered; the objective is to discover a topical localization for any abnormality that is uncovered. Thus, a defect must be explored enough to determine if it is compatible with glaucoma (arcuate, nasal step), optic neuropathy (arcuate, central scotoma), chiasmal disease (bitemporal hemianopia, junctional), or a retrochiasmal process (homonymous hemianopia). Quantitation is necessary so a subtle abnormality can be detected or so the field can be followed for progression. Static threshold testing is required to obtain this quantitative data.

Each patient for whom formal visual field testing is contemplated for a neuro-ophthalmic examination has different requirements for level of testing required and different capacities to undergo testing. Indeed, there may be limitations of available equipment or expertise in the office. For most patients who are fully cooperative, there is little reason to deviate from the standard office routine of quantitative static threshold testing in both eyes. If an abnormality is discovered, the information is usually sufficient to make a typical diagnosis or at least to indicate the direction for further testing. If follow-up is contemplated, it can be done without the necessity for repeat testing to establish a quantitative baseline, as would have been required if the first test had been a suprathreshold screening pattern.

For patients who are not fully alert or cooperative, a decision must be made whether to attempt quantitative testing. If it is not likely that serial follow-up of the field will be required, a suprathreshold screening test is probably a more appropriate choice. The density of the test pattern and the attendant time requirement must be tailored to the patient's concentration abilities.

If there are technicians available who are skilled in Goldmann perimetry, many patients who are unable to complete quantitative static threshold testing can perform acceptably with this method. *Just because an office acquires an automated perimeter does not mean it should discard the apparatus previously used!*

Either before or after an automated visual field has been performed, suspicion may be raised that the patient has functional, rather than organic, visual loss. In such an event, the testing must be moved from the automated perimeter to the tangent screen. Functional patients perform poorly at automated perimetry, but there is no consistent abnormality that is pathognomonic. At the tangent screen, however, a number of characteristic patterns of functional visual loss can be appreciated. Even if an office does not have a black felt screen and a set of test objects, tangent testing can be performed using a blank wall, a movable chair for patients, and an aspirin tablet glued to a wand.

■ Peripheral versus Central Visual Field Testing

In most offices with the capability, automated static perimetry within the central 30 degrees is the routine test performed when visual fields are ordered. Fortunately, most field defects of neuro-ophthalmic significance are manifest within this central zone. Although they may be more obvious in the periphery, hemianopic defects almost always demonstrate a step along the vertical meridian centrally. Nonglaucomatous optic neuropathies share with glaucoma a tendency to produce central visual field defects. Thus, testing limited to the central 30 degrees will miss only a small percentage of defects. It should be understood, however, that the peripheral sparing associated with ring scotomas of retinal degeneration and sparing of the monocular temporal crescent in occipital lobe disease will be missed unless peripheral testing is performed in addition to the standard central test. Peripheral testing, even if it is a rapid suprathreshold screen, can add useful diagnostic confirmation to a suspected abnormality on the central test.

■ Selection of an Automated Test

Taking the foregoing factors into account, the following are recommendations for testing in various circumstances.

Quantitative Testing

The Humphrey 30-2, Octopus 32 or 38, or an equivalent static threshold central test, in which point locations are offset from the vertical and horizontal meridian, should be used so that steps can be detected. If peripheral field information is desirable either because of suspected abnormality of the central test or clinical indication, the central test can be supplemented with a Humphrey peripheral-68, Octopus 07, or an equivalent peripheral suprathreshold screening program.

Screening for Diagnosis

If patients cannot be expected to complete quantitative testing, a Humphrey 120 full-field, Octopus 07, or equivalent suprathreshold screening program covering the field to 60 degrees with at least 100 points may be selected. A threshold-related strategy with retesting of missed points using maximum intensity stimuli (three-zone test) provides optimal information.

Screening for Abnormalities

Patients who cannot tolerate screening for diagnosis but who are able to cooperate for shorter automated tests are not commonly encountered. Tests screening 40 points can be used, but quick Goldmann perimetry using a V-4e stimulus, tangent screen testing, or color confrontation may be just as reliable.

■ Interpretation of the Automated Visual Field

Clinicians often express dismay at the difficulty in interpreting the results of automated perimetry because they are so comfortable interpreting charts derived from manual kinetic perimetry. Goldmann perimetry is usually performed by trained technicians who filter out ambiguous or contradictory patient responses before they plot the charts that are shown to ophthalmologists. Automated perimeters do not do this; rather, they dutifully record all patient responses whether "valid" or not valid. Most of the time, the difficulty interpreting automated fields results from this noise in the data as much as from unfamiliarity with the data presentation format.

■ Patient Reliability Parameters

Most automated perimeters monitor patient reliability. They do not do so continuously, however, nor do they listen to patient complaints. So the machine-generated reliability parameters are not to be considered a substitute for technician evaluation of patient cooperation, which needs to be recorded manually on the visual field chart at the conclusion of the examination.

Each patient's fixation stability during the test should be continuously observed by technicians on the video display or through the observation periscope. In addition, the perimeter will periodically display a bright stimulus inside the expected location of the physiological blind spot. If patients respond to the stimulus, a fixation loss is recorded. The sum of the fixation losses divided by the number of such trials is a measure of fixation reliability. Care must be taken to ensure that the "expected" location of the physiological blind spot is accurate. The patient's head may have moved slightly since the test began, moving the physiological blind spot to a different position in the perimeter bowl away from the location of the periodic blind spot check stimuli. If this possibility is not continuously monitored by technicians and readjustments made as necessary, the fixation losses may be recorded as high although the patient has excellent fixation.

The perimeter may also monitor reliability in two other respects. False-positive trials are presented when the machine makes all the preparatory motor sounds and delays that it usually does prior to stimulus presentation, but a stimulus does not appear. If patients respond, a false-positive response is recorded. The sum of these responses divided by the number of such trials is recorded on the chart. For false-negative trials, the machine presents a bright stimulus at a location where a stimulus was previously seen by the patient. If patients fail to respond, a false-negative response is recorded. The sum of these responses divided by the number of such trials is recorded on the chart.

These three fractions constitute the most frequently used patient reliability parameters. High fixation losses, not related to patient positioning errors, and high false-negative results are indications that the visual field quality is suboptimal, but characteristic visual field defect patterns can usually be identified in spite of poor patient reliability. High false-positive values, however, indicating a "trigger-happy" patient, can totally obscure complete hemianopic defects, so the field result is invalidated.

■ The Printout

In threshold visual field testing, the stimulus brightness that is seen 50% of the time at each point is estimated. Sometimes stimulus strength is recorded in physical terms, or apostilbs, but usually a logarithmic scale with decibel units is used. The brightest stimulus available on a given perimeter is arbitrarily assigned a value of 0 decibels, and progressively dimmer stimuli are assigned larger numbers. A convenient way to view a *numeric printout* of threshold values is to think of larger numbers as better retinal sensitivity.

The *gray scale printout* assigns progressively darker shades of gray to progressively lower thresholds. All zero-decibel thresholds are printed black. Of course, threshold is usually measured only at 80 or fewer locations, so the gray scale printout assumes, or interpolates, the threshold values between measured points. As will be appreciated in reviewing the illustrations in this chapter, interpolation can be inconvenient when attempting to evaluate whether a step is aligned along the vertical meridian.

The *difference printout* is a set of results from subtraction of the "normal" threshold from the patient's threshold at each tested point. The normal threshold is usually an age-corrected value that was derived empirically and stored in the perimeter memory. In some perimeters without stored normative values, however, the "normal" threshold is really an "expected" value calculated from the patient's own test results. Scanning a difference printout for large values helps to pinpoint the most abnormal areas of each patient's visual field.

In the Humphrey perimeter Statpac (Allergan–Humphrey, San Leandro, CA) software, the difference printout is reformatted according to the statistical likelihood that a patient's threshold at each point is normal. As in the gray scale, the darker symbols indicate a more abnormal result, indicating a slim likelihood that the point is normal.

■ The Vertical Meridian

The importance of the vertical meridian in neuro-ophthalmic diagnosis cannot be overemphasized. The signature of a hemianopic defect, seen with lesions of the visual pathways at or anywhere posterior to the chiasm, is alignment along the vertical meridian. This alignment will be manifest as a step off in sensitivity across at least a portion of the vertical meridian.

Unfortunately, in automated perimetry this "vertical step" can sometimes be difficult to detect unless specific focus is directed toward the vertical meridian during interpretation. Several factors may conspire to make a true vertical step obscure.

1. A normal decrease in retinal sensitivity may occur across the superior visual field, crossing the vertical meridian, making both sides of the superior field dark on the gray scale.
2. The step may be subtle, so that the gray shading on one side of the vertical meridian is only slightly darker than on the other. In some cases, the step may be within a single shade of gray and be detectable only by reference to the numeric plot.
3. Patients may be marginally reliable, causing inconsistencies in the observations across the vertical meridian.
4. Normal fluctuation in visual field determinations may obscure a real step or produce an apparent step when one is not present.

What sort of special attention should be accorded the vertical meridian during interpretation? The following strategies should be employed, especially when the clinical circumstances suggest that a lesion at or posterior to the chiasm may be present. (1) The gray scale should be scanned for a step across the vertical meridian. (2) The numeric plot should always be scrutinized, because the gray scale can be misleading. Each threshold value on one side should be compared with the corresponding value on the other side of the vertical meridian. The most important comparisons involve the pairs of thresholds immediately adjacent to the vertical meridian, but should also include the pairs from the second columns away. At least three adjacent pairs should show a step in the same direction to suggest a significant step (i.e., the higher thresholds should all be on one side of the vertical meridian and the lower thresholds on the other). (3) If a step is detected, attention should then be directed to the field of the patient's other eye. Lesions at or behind the chiasm will produce a defect in the fellow eye, which usually will also show alignment along the vertical meridian. Some patients have defects in the fellow eye, such as blindness or a central scotoma, that do not align along the vertical, but these junctional defects have localizing value to the anterior chiasm. Indeed, strictly monocular (the field of the fellow eye is normal) temporal defects that align along the vertical meridian occur with lesions of the prechiasmal intracranial optic nerve, but they also occur in other optic neuropathies such as glaucoma and transiently in optic neuritis. When a vertical step is observed in *only one eye,* it is wise to retain suspicion of a central lesion but with the understanding that an intracranial lesion is far less likely than if a vertical step had been detected in both eyes.

If clinicians are uncertain whether a vertical step is present, consideration should be given to either repeating the test or to running a quick retest of the area of interest. A custom threshold test with a cluster of 9 to 16 points straddling the vertical meridian centered on the area of interest should be performed. With this additional information, a decision whether a true step is present can often be made.

■ Statistical Aids to Visual Field Interpretation

An extensive discussion of the software enhancement packages available for statistical analysis of visual field data from automated perimeters is beyond the scope of this chapter, mainly because the packages are specifically designed for detecting and following glaucoma. Their principal neuro-ophthalmic application is in detecting and following other subtle optic neuropathies, such as early optic nerve decompensation in papilledema or dysthyroid ophthalmopathy. In these clinical settings, a "statistical" result that indicates early damage or progression is usually just as valid for other optic neuropathies as it is for glaucoma. In other neuro-ophthalmic conditions, however, especially those producing hemianopias, the statistical analysis software as currently configured is not helpful.

■ Topographic Localization of Visual Field Defects

The Optic Nerve

There is only limited anatomical variability in the optic nerve, but, unfortunately, there is often enormous variability in perimetry when testing the field of a diseased optic nerve. Seldom is one discrete area of the nerve damaged and the rest totally spared. Most optic neuropathies produce a generalized reduction in optic nerve function with characteristic focal damage superimposed on it. This variability, or fluctuation, may in an individual test blur the borders of arcuate scotomas, make a central scotoma seem to have hemianopic characteristics, or obscure the alignment of a defect along the vertical or horizontal meridians. Topographic localization thus remains an inexact art. Occasionally, localizing visual field characteristics may appear to be present, when in fact they are not (or would not be on repeat testing) and lead to further testing for an incorrect differential diagnosis. At other times, typical defects may be obscured (and would not be on repeat testing) and fail to point clinicians in the proper diagnostic direction. It is therefore a good rule to repeat the visual field test if there is any question of the validity of the result.

Field defects caused by nonglaucomatous optic neuropathies tend to have a different appearance on manual kinetic and automated static threshold perimetry. On an automated field, generalized depression of sensitivity with an abnormal mean defect corresponds to peripheral constriction of isopters on Goldmann perimetry. Arcuate nerve fiber layer defects will not generally be as defined with sharp edges on automated printouts as on a drawing of a manual kinetic field. Experience with identification of characteristic field patterns on manual charts is of considerable value in detecting the same patterns on automated fields where they may be obscured by fluctuation or generalized depression.

If an arcuate or nasal step defect appears, the lesion is likely to be at the optic disc (Fig 1). If the defect is altitudinal, either retinal vascular disease or optic disc pathology is likely. Central and cecocentral defects are most likely retrobulbar optic nerve or macular in origin (Fig 2). Monocular temporal hemianopia is characteristic of intracranial optic nerve pathology (Fig 3). Paracentral scotomas, generalized depression, and focal peripheral depression are not localizing.

The Optic Chiasm

The two optic nerves, after leaving the optic canals, run posteriorly and superiorly at an angle of 45 degrees to the horizontal to come together in the midline at the optic chiasm. Because of this angulation, the undersurface of the chiasm is usually as much as a centimeter above the top surface of the pituitary gland, explaining why pituitary tumors must be quite large to compress the chiasm. The anteroposterior location of the chiasm is quite variable: It may lie in front of, directly over, or behind the pituitary gland. This variable location makes the task of predicting anatomical relationships based on examination of the visual field dangerous.

Despite these caveats, the signature of chiasmal disease is bitemporal hemianopia, and the presence of this field defect is a reliable indication of a problem localized to the chiasm. Fortunately, it is no longer necessary to attempt to be specific about localization within the chiasm because once bitemporal hemianopia is detected neuroimaging of the chiasmal area will provide the needed specificity (Figs 4, 5).

Unfortunately, classic bitemporal hemianopia continues to be misdiagnosed, most commonly as optic neuritis or macular degeneration, because of the doctor's failure to perform visual fields. Accordingly, a high level of suspicion for chiasmal disease must accompany evaluation of patients with unexplained visual loss, optic atrophy, or obscure visual complaint. Attention to the

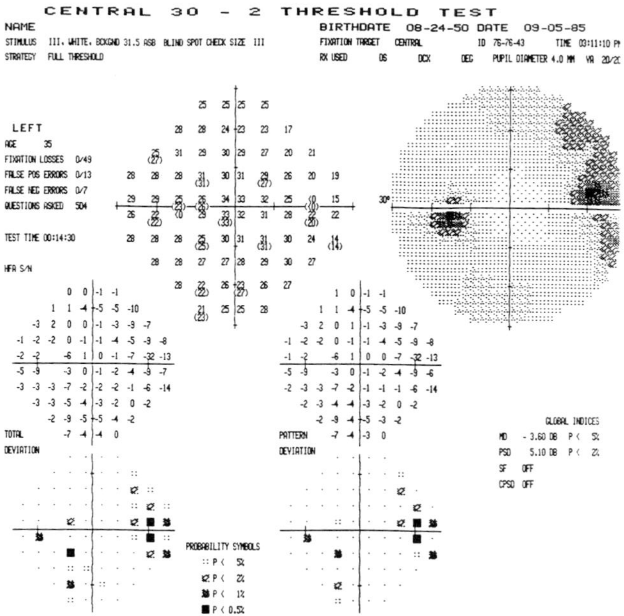

A

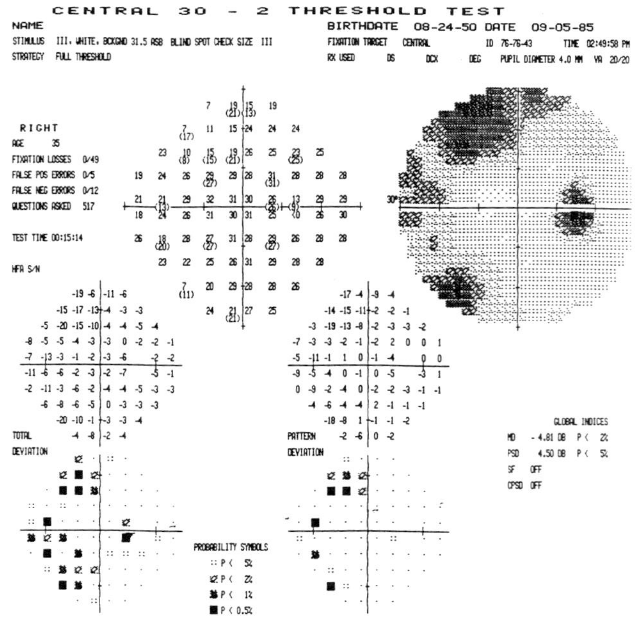

B

Figure 1 *Humphrey 30-2 visual fields of a 35-year-old woman with pseudotumor cerebri and bilateral severe papilledema. Nasal visual field depression occurs more in the right eye (B) than in the left eye (A). No consistent step along the vertical meridian is identifiable. After normalization of the intracranial pressure, these field defects resolved. Top row, left: patient reliability parameters. Top row, middle: actual threshold estimates, in decibels* (dB)*. Second threshold determination at each point is in parentheses. Top row, right: gray scale. Darker shading reflects lower threshold values. Middle row, left: total deviation numeric plot. Age-corrected normal threshold values are subtracted from patient's threshold values at each point. Middle row, middle: pattern deviation numeric plot. Values in total deviation plot are adjusted by a constant value to compensate for any overall reduction of sensitivity. Middle row, right: on some printouts, the results of a glaucoma hemifield test are reported, not relevant to neuro-ophthalmic diagnosis. Bottom row, left: total deviation probability plot. Darker symbols indicate less probability that the point is normal. Bottom row, middle: pattern deviation probability plot. After compensation for any overall reduction of sensitivity, the darker symbols denote points that are worse than others. Bottom row, right: visual field indices.* MD = *mean deviation (from normal);* PSD = *pattern standard deviation;* SF = *short-term fluctuation;* CPSD = *corrected pattern standard deviation.*

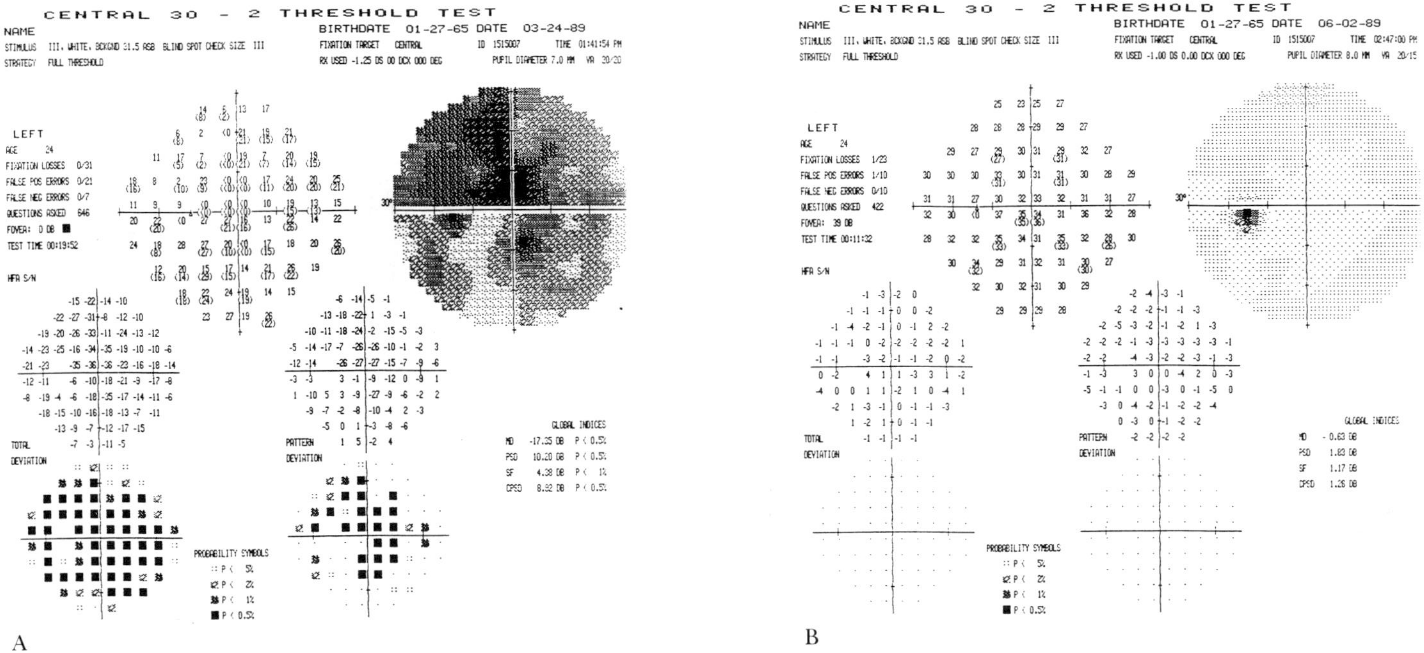

Figure 2 *Humphrey 30-2 visual fields of a 34-year-old woman with optic neuritis, left eye. The right visual acuity and field (not shown) was normal. The left eye had 20/20 visual acuity, but the field (A) shows a dense scotoma and a measured foveal sensitivity of 0 decibels* (dB). *Alignment along the vertical meridian disappeared on left eye visual field testing six months later (B), when acuity had recovered to 20/15. See Figure 1 for row-by-row explanation*

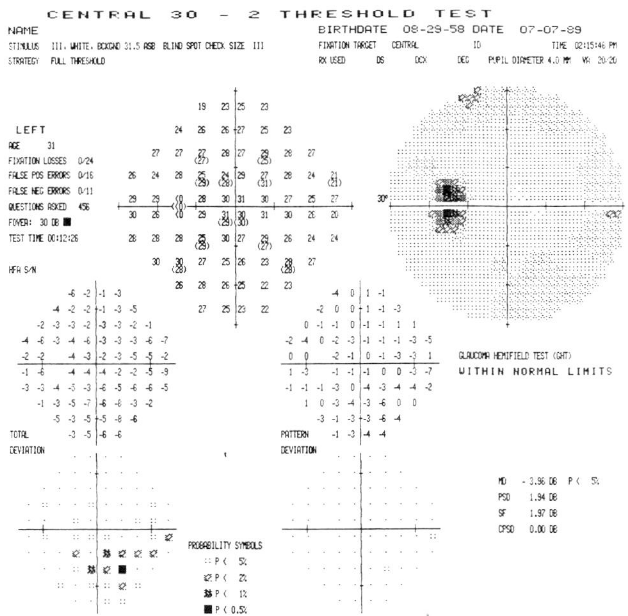

A

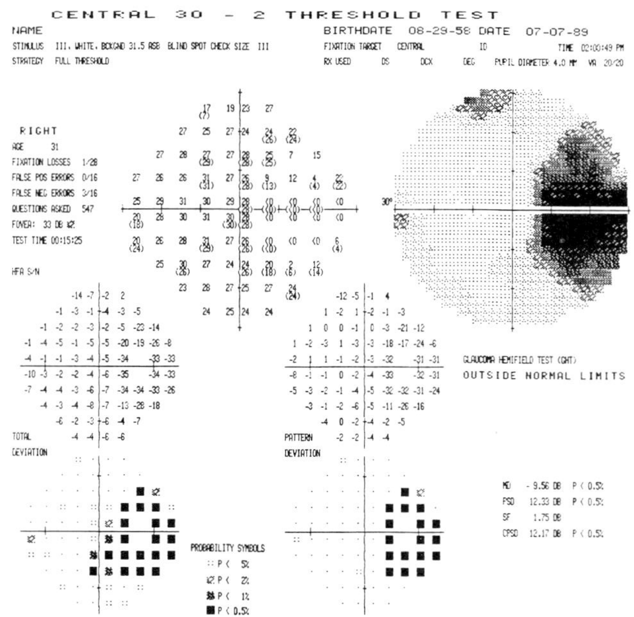

B

Figure 3 *Humphrey 30-2 visual fields of a 30-year-old physician who noted recent onset of a visual field defect and mild visual blurring, right eye. The 20/20 right eye had a dense scotoma contiguous with the physiological blind spot (B). The 20/20 left eye has mild generalized depression (mean deviation = −3.96 dB), but the field is otherwise normal (A). A large arachnoid cyst compressed the right optic nerve intracranially anterior to the chiasm, resulting in this monocular temporal defect, which did not align along the vertical meridian. See Figure 1 for row-by-row explanation.*

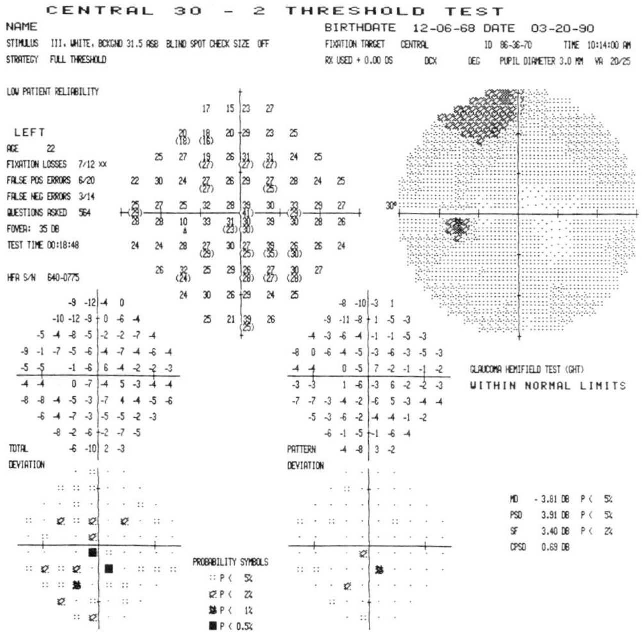

A

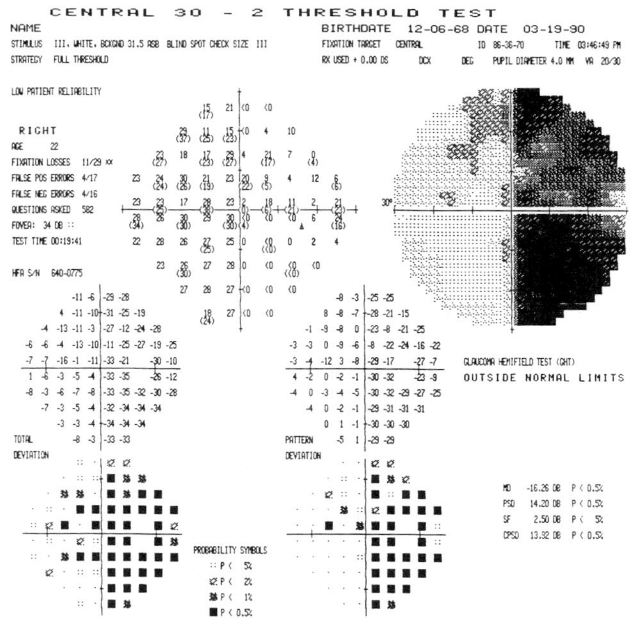

B

Figure 4 *Humphrey 30-2 visual fields of a 21-year-old woman several months after severe closed head injury. Visual acuity in her right eye was 20/30, and the visual field shows a striking incomplete temporal defect respecting the vertical meridian (B). The 20/25 left eye looks deceptively normal on the gray scale, but reference to the numeric display shows a step across the vertical meridian involving all 5 pairs of points in the superior field (A). In spite of very poor reliability parameters, it is possible to detect this grossly asymmetrical bitemporal hemianopsia. It was associated with a relative afferent pupillary defect in the right eye and mild right optic atrophy. Computed tomographic scanning showed multiple fractures at the skull base. The clinical diagnosis was chiasmal contusion. See Figure 1 for row-by-row explanation.*

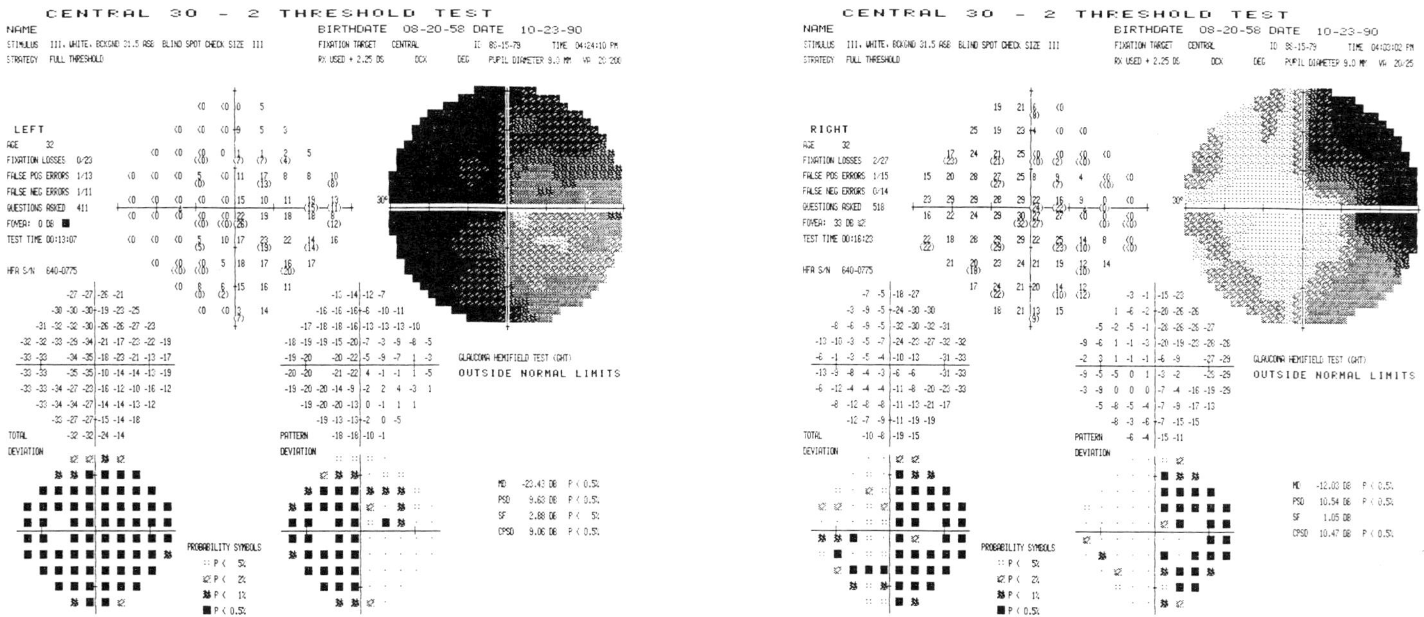

A   B

Figure 5 *Humphrey 30-2 visual fields of a 32-year-old man who noted headaches and blurred vision with gradual loss of his axillary hair. Right eye was 20/25 with an incomplete temporal hemianopia and some mild depression in the nasal field (B). The left eye was 20/200 with generalized visual field depression that was absolute at many points in the temporal field (including the fovea) and showed a consistent step along the vertical meridian (A). Color vision was depressed, left worse than right eye, but there was no afferent pupillary defect. Computed tomographic scanning showed a large pituitary adenoma with chiasmal compression. See Figure 1 for row-by-row explanation.*

possibility of partial bitemporal hemianopia, with careful attention to the vertical meridian during interpretation, affords the best protection against missed diagnosis.

Retrochiasmal Visual Pathways

Posterior to the optic chiasm, visual information from the right hemifield of both eyes is carried by the left visual pathway, and the information from the left hemifield of both eyes travels in the right visual pathway. Lesions of structures posterior to the chiasm, with one very rare exception, produce defects in both eyes on the same side of the visual field: a homonymous hemianopia. Because it is possible to have 20/20 vision using the macular fibers from only one hemifield, lesions affecting only one side are not associated with defective visual acuity. Performance and interpretation of visual fields must emphasize the search for alignment of any defects along the vertical meridian. Just as in chiasmal disease, so called respect for the vertical is a critically important diagnostic feature.

Retinal fibers from the two eyes, which transmit information about the same point in the visual field, become gradually juxtaposed as the visual pathways travel posteriorly toward the visual cortex. Field defects from posterior lesions are very similar if not superimposable in the two eyes. This phenomenon is known as congruity. By contrast, lesions just posterior to the chiasm in the optic tracts tend to be quite noncongruous.

A complete homonymous hemianopia, however, affecting the entire hemifield in both eyes, does not have localizing significance (Fig 6). If a lesion is severe enough to produce a total loss of function in the visual pathway of one side, hemianopia will be complete no matter where in the visual pathway the lesion occurs. To avoid the common error of trying to localize a complete homonymous hemianopia, it is best to remember that congruity of the field defect is a useful concept only for incomplete hemianopias (Figs 7–9).

Functional Visual Loss

In patients with functional visual loss, no organic disease or objective confirmation can be found to explain the results attained with subjective tests such as visual acuity or visual fields. The process may be unconscious, in which patients have no awareness of the psychological basis of the problem (as in hysteria), or it may be under conscious control, as in malingering to obtain compensation for alleged injury.

An automated threshold perimeter affords inadequate spatial or temporal orientation to functional patients, so characteristic patterns of field loss do not usually emerge. Most commonly, severe generalized field depression with poor reliability parameters and high short-term fluctuation is seen, but there is nothing specific to implicate a functional process. Only a high index of suspicion based on a mismatch of objective and subjective findings will cause clinicians to repeat the field at the tangent screen to obtain the correct diagnosis.

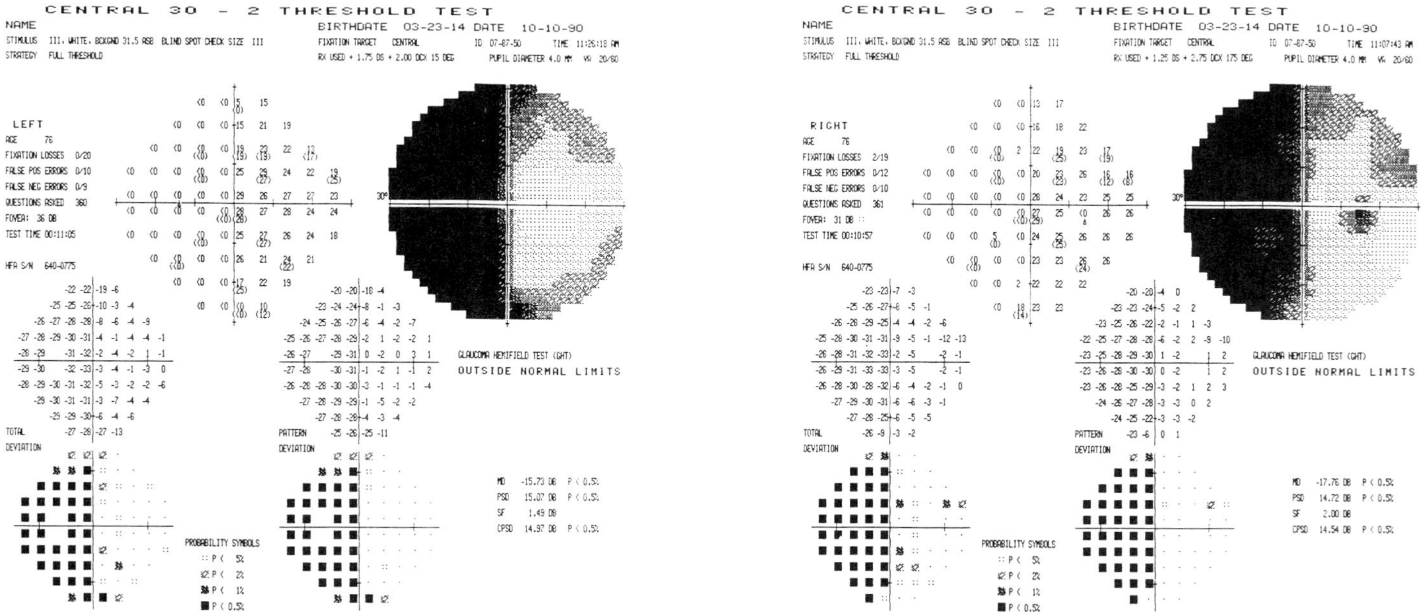

A B

Figure 6 *Humphrey 30-2 visual fields of a 76-year-old man on anticoagulant therapy who had sudden headache and left hemiparesis. Visual acuity was 20/60 in each eye, and there was a complete left homonymous hemianopia. (B) Right eye and (A) left eye. Alignment along the vertical meridian was not perfect, probably due to testing artifacts, because the field defect to confrontation was absolute and limited to the left hemifields. Such complete homonymous hemianopias have no localizing significance. Computed tomographic scanning disclosed a large right temporal hematoma. See Figure 1 for row-by-row explanation.*

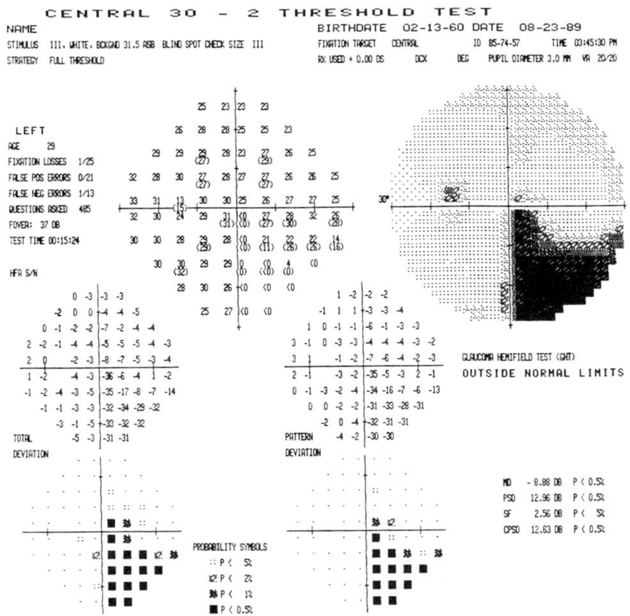

A

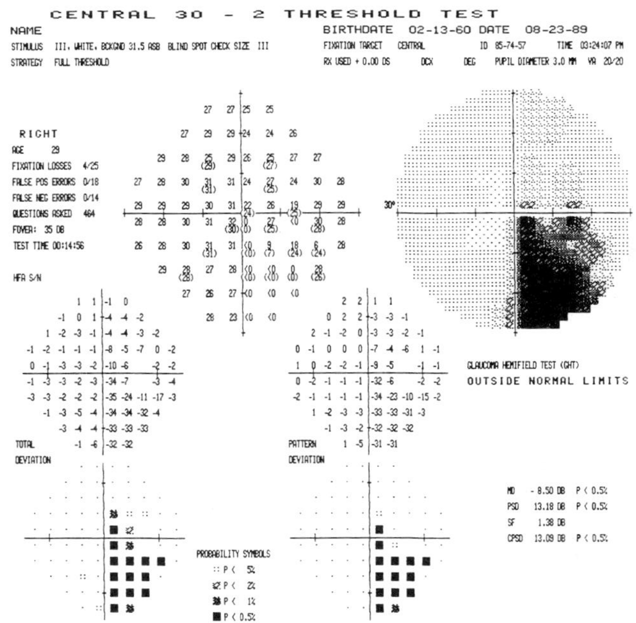

B

Figure 7 *Humphrey 30-2 visual fields of a 29-year-old patient with a glioblastoma of the left posterolateral thalamus and adjacent visual radiations. The visual acuity was 20/20 in each eye. The right eye (B) shows a dense inferior wedge-shaped scotoma partly separated from the physiological blind spot. The left eye (A) demonstrates noncongruity in the nasal periphery. The alignment along the vertical meridian is excellent. See Figure 1 for row-by-row explanation.*

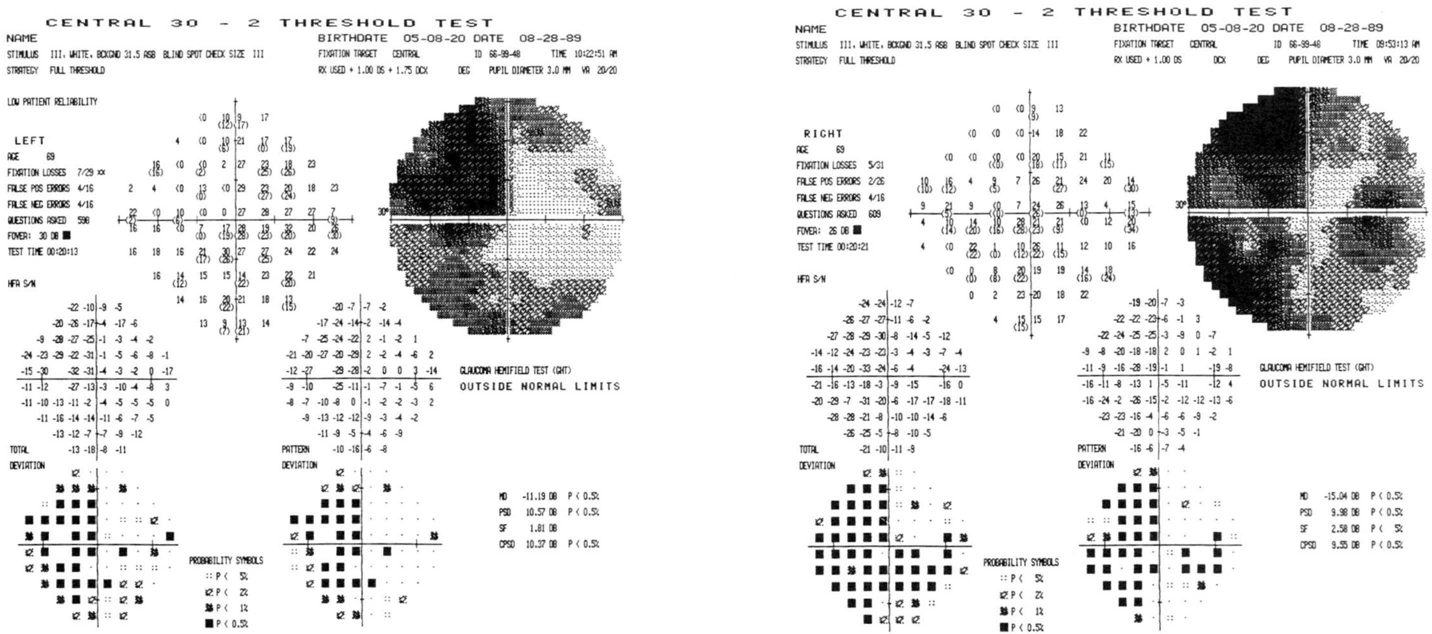

A

B

Figure 8 *Humphrey 30-2 visual fields of a 69-year-old patient who suffered a right parietal ischemic stroke with left hemiparesis. Patient reliability parameters are poor, perhaps accounting for the patchy involvement of both eyes, but a noncongruous left homonymous hemianopsia is present. (B) Right eye and (A) left eye. See Figure 1 for row-by-row explanation.*

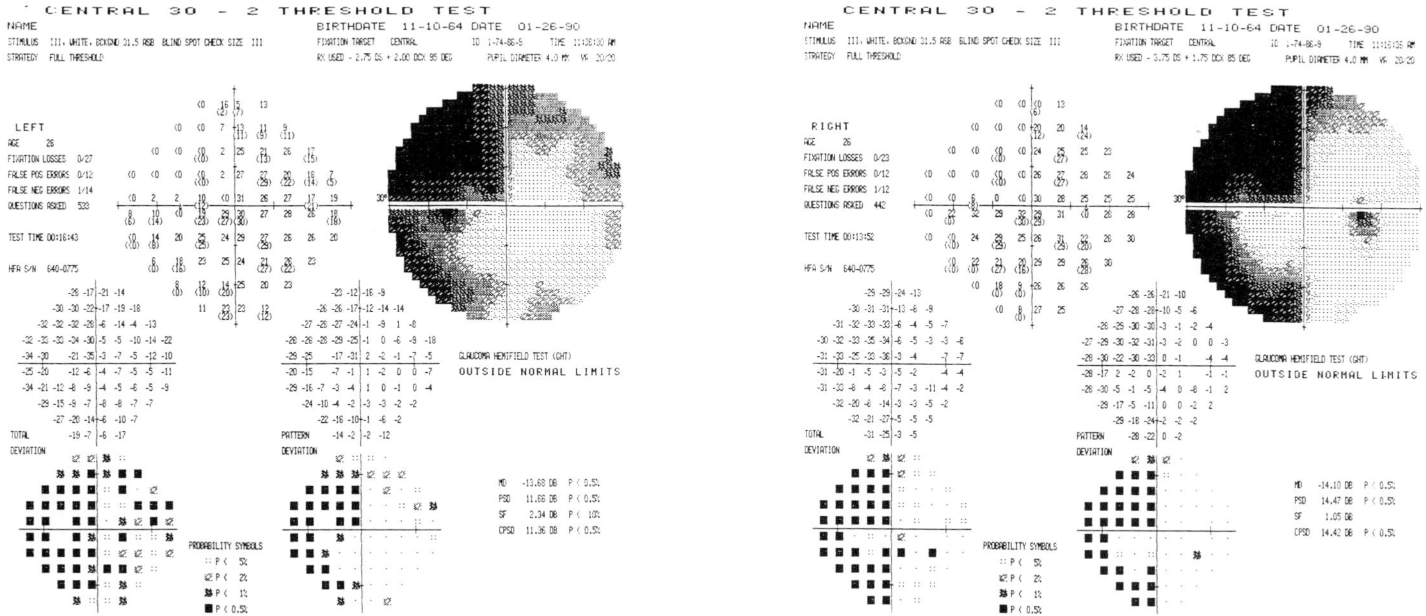

A B

Figure 9 *Humphrey 30-2 visual fields of an asymptomatic 25-year-old man with a lesion of the right calcarine cortex thought to represent infarction. The field defects of right (B) and left (A) eyes are reasonably congruous, consisting of a nearly absolute left superior quadrantanopia plus a crescent-shaped defect of the left inferior field. See Figure 1 for row-by-row explanation.*

■ Summary

The automated perimeter presents new challenges to clinicians comfortable with the use of the Goldmann perimeter in neuro-ophthalmic diagnosis. An understanding of the basic differences between kinetic and static threshold perimetry, an intelligent choice of automated test programs, and an interpretive strategy focusing on the vertical meridian will result in optimal use of this important technological advance.

Optic Nerve Sheath Decompression: History, Techniques, and Indications

Robert C. Sergott, M.D.

Historical Perspective

Although most ophthalmologists, including glaucoma subspecialists and neuro-ophthalmologists, receive similar training, subscribe to (and hopefully read) the same journals, and attend many of the same scientific meetings, a diversity of opinion exists concerning the management of various optic neuropathies. Glaucoma, the most common optic neuropathy, frequently is treated surgically. Ophthalmologists, including glaucoma subspecialists, have little difficulty recommending surgery as a rational form of management. Inherent in accepting surgery in appropriate circumstances is a belief that pressure on axons and blood vessels may damage optic nerve function.

In contrast, neuro-ophthalmologists, perhaps because of a more medical/neurological orientation, have accepted surgical management primarily for extrinsic compression of the optic nerve, such as orbital neoplasms and dysthyroid optic neuropathy. Neuro-ophthalmologists, as a group, have generally used medical therapy, particularly corticosteroids, in treating visual loss associated with "intrinsic" optic neuropathies such as papilledema, anterior ischemic optic neuropathy (AION), and inflammatory optic neuritis. As a result, patients often receive massive amounts of steroids despite uncertainty about proven therapeutic effect and despite well-known, potentially fatal complications.

Optic nerve surgery was proposed over a century ago by DeWecker [1] and Carter [2], yet this therapeutic alternative (specifically optic nerve sheath decompression [ONSD] or fenestration [ONSF]), has not been widely accepted by neuro-ophthalmologists. To dare suggest that ONSD could be appropriate treatment risked "excommunication" by the high priests of the subspecialty.

In spite of experimental and limited clinical success with ONSD [3–6], the procedure was used infrequently. Its resurgence as a form of treatment for intrinsic optic nerve disease should be credited in part to the advent of high resolution computed tomographic (CT) scans. These axial and coronal images in patients with increased intracranial pressures and vision-threatening papilledema demonstrated unequivocal expansion of the subarachnoid space of the optic nerve (Fig 1). At approximately the same time, patients with pseudotu-

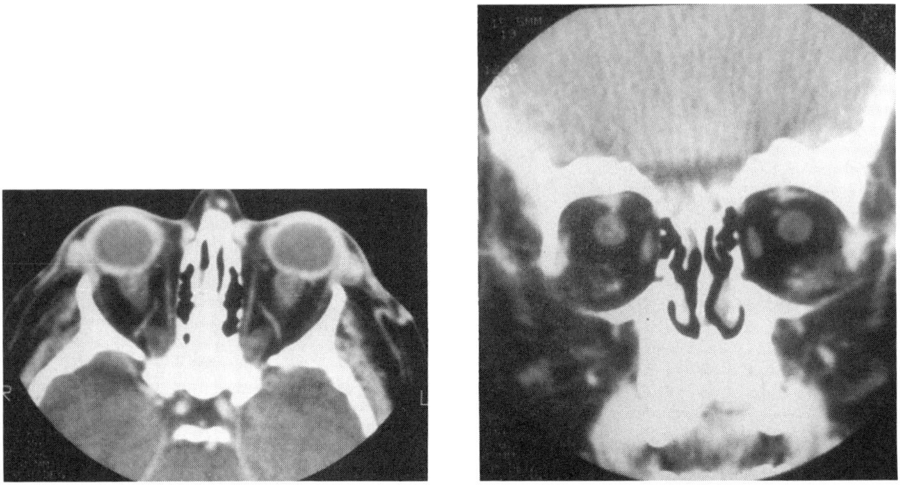

A B

Figure 1 *Expanded subarachnoid space of intraorbital optic nerves due to pseudotumor cerebri demonstrated by axial (A) and coronal (B) computed tomographic scans. Enlargement of the optic nerve sheath complexes is not always this dramatic, and relatively normal neuroimaging studies should not deter surgical intervention.*

mor cerebri were reported in whom profound visual loss developed despite functioning lumboperitoneal shunts [7, 8]. These neuroradiological and clinical observations prompted a reassessment of local pressure phenomena in chronic papilledema. I review the surgical techniques for ONSD and describe the currently accepted indications for the procedure as well as its controversial use in certain diseases.

■ Surgical Technique

General Considerations

Patients and surgeons must understand explicitly that ONSD may permanently blind the operated eye. The risk of such a disastrous complication in our experience of 300 operations is 1%. Therefore, ONSD should be considered only when maximal medical therapy has failed or when the natural history of the disease is such that delay in surgical intervention will result in irreversible, significant optic nerve damage.

We advocate general anesthesia for all patients because the traction exerted on the globe and orbital structures produces too much pain to be controlled by local anesthesia. In addition, we always apply a light patch and plastic shield over the closed, unoperated eye. Because ONSD is frequently performed on the eye with the most impaired visual function, inadvertent, intraoperative pressure on the contralateral eye by a member of the surgical team could be catastrophic.

The orbital area to be operated on is prepared and draped in the usual sterile manner. A wrist rest, identical to that used in vitreoretinal surgery, is also used.

Surgeons must approach the optic nerve with the same precision and care used in clipping intracranial aneurysms and in resecting epidural spinal cord tumors. Excessive stretching, torsion, and traction of the optic nerve can produce permanent blindness. A thorough understanding of orbital anatomy, especially the vasculature of the optic nerve, is mandatory.

Medial Approach

Two approaches—the medial transconjunctival and lateral Kronlein-Berke orbitotomies—have been used for ONSD [9, 10]. No controlled studies have been undertaken to recommend the medial or lateral approach.

We prefer the medial approach because this technique allows the nerve to be isolated more easily and avoids removal of the lateral bony orbital wall. In patients with eyes set deeply in the orbit and in patients with high myopia, exposure of the optic nerve may be more difficult. We have not encountered a patient, however, in whom surgical exposure was inadequate.

A wire Barraquer speculum opens the lids, and a lateral canthotomy is performed to provide more space in the operative field and to allow additional space for retrobulbar postoperative swelling.

Conjunctiva is incised with blunt-tipped Westcott scissors three and one-half mm posterior to the medial limbus. The distance for the incision is measured with calipers to avoid cutting the medial rectus. The conjunctival incision is extended superiorly and inferiorly for 270 degrees, sparing the area around the lateral rectus.

The quadrants between the medial rectus and vertical rectus muscles are opened with sharp and blunt dissection using curved Stevens scissors. With a Gass muscle hook, 4-0 black silk traction sutures are placed under the superior and inferior rectus muscles.

The medial rectus muscle is isolated and cleaned free of its fascial attachments. After a 6-0 Vicryl suture double-armed with S-29 needles is weaved through the medial rectus near its insertion and locked on itself at the superior and inferior poles of the muscle, the muscle is detached from the globe with Abli scissors. A small "stump" of muscle tendon (approximately 1 mm) is left on the globe.

This tendon stump is used to place a "baseball stitch" traction suture through the entire length of the previous insertion of the medial rectus. The "bites" of the suture are relatively close together and resemble the laces of a baseball. A 6-0 Vicryl suture double-armed with S-29 needles is used for the baseball stitch. To place this suture, the globe is fixated with 0.12-mm forceps, and the belly of the needle is positioned on the thinnest sclera immediately behind the insertion (often the bluish color of the choroid is visible in this area). The point of the needle is then engaged beneath the stump and advanced forward. This portion of the procedure is done with the operating microscope. The intrascleral course of the needle should be seen at all times. Just anterior to the muscle insertion, the scleral thickness increases to 0.8 mm (compared to 0.3 mm just posterior to the insertion). It is important that the suture engage sclera and not merely episclera. Each bite of the baseball stitch covers a length of 1.0 to 2.0 mm. We have found that the baseball stitch is essential to obtain adequate exposure of the optic nerve.

If bleeding occurs after removal of the medial rectus, we apply light, wet field bipolar cautery anterior to the stump. We avoid cauterizing directly on the stump because shrinkage of the stump by cautery makes placement of the baseball stitch much more difficult.

The globe is then elevated and abducted using the baseball stitch and the sutures under the vertical rectus muscles. The intrascleral course of the long posterior ciliary artery (LPCA) is then identified. The LPCA is the critical landmark for maintaining orientation of the optic nerve and lies midway between the superior and inferior poles of the medial rectus insertion. The LPCA course is a ridge in the sclera that may be slightly pigmented and may be identified in approximately 80% of eyes. In the remaining 20%, surgeons must keep the eye oriented in the 3- to 9-o'clock axis and must perform the procedure between the two medial vortex veins. Meticulous orientation of the globe is mandatory to isolate the optic nerve in an atraumatic fashion.

During elevation and abduction of the globe, the size of the pupil is monitored constantly. If the pupil dilates more than 2 mm in diameter, the eye should be returned promptly to normal anatomical position. Several mechanisms may account for intraoperative pupillary dilation. The iris and the ciliary nerves may be ischemic. We believe that this mechanism occurs when pupillary dilation is asymmetric.

When concentric pupillary dilation occurs, intraoperative angle closure glaucoma or choroidal detachments have been observed in three cases (see Complications). In this case, the globe becomes quite firm as opposed to the usual situation when traction on the globe produces relative hypotonia.

The most important and most frequent reason for pupillary dilation is probably ischemia to the retina and optic nerve. Because the contralateral eye is occluded with a patch and shield, patients are monocular, and if the operated eye has "no light perception" vision, then pupillary dilation will occur. Therefore, we use the size of the pupil as an intraoperative visually evoked response and as a gauge of perfusion of the optic nerve and retina.

The posterior reflection of Tenon's capsule holding the orbital fat posteriorly is then lysed with blunt dissection using cotton-tipped applicators. In older patients, this membrane may be absent or quite diaphanous. In young patients, however, it is quite thick and requires sharp dissection with Westcott or transsphenoidal scissors.

The LPCA leads directly to the optic nerve. After the reflection of Tenon's capsule has been lysed, orbital fat migrates anteriorly. The fat is maneuvered with a Fischer malleable retractor in the medial orbit and with cotton-tipped applicators (Fig 2). In patients with chronic optic nerve edema, adhesions form between the meninges and orbital fat. These adhesions are gently lysed by manipulating the Stevens tenotomy hook between the nerve and fat. In breaking these adhesions, caution must be used to avoid tearing the posterior ciliary arteries. The optic nerve is isolated between the applicators, and the ciliary vessels are gently twisted out of the operative field with the applicators to expose a relatively avascular area of the meningeal sheath (Fig 3).

The dura is incised boldly with a long-handled tympanic membrane blade, frequently used by vitreoretinal surgeons to make sclerotomies (Fig 4). The

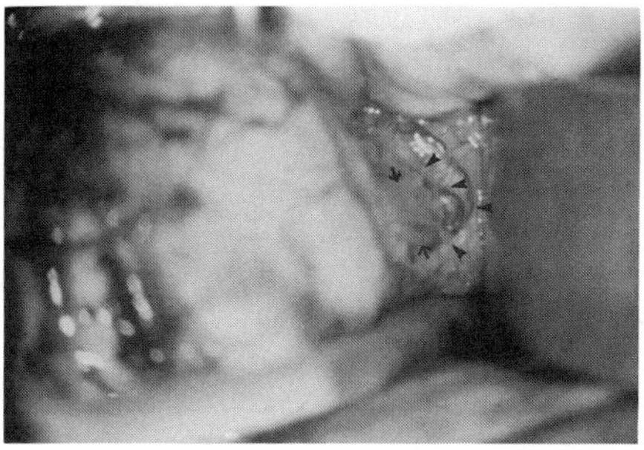

Figure 2 *Optic nerve* (arrows) *encased within adhesions between its meningeal cover and orbital fat* (arrowheads). *These adhesions must be dissected from the nerve before optic nerve sheath decompression is performed. These adhesions occur when papilledema has been long-standing.*

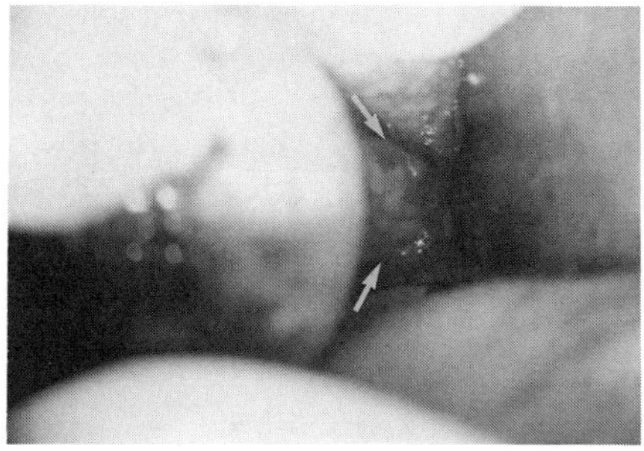

Figure 3 *Optic nerve illustrated in Figure 2 that has been isolated from the surrounding orbital fat, and the posterior ciliary arteries have been retracted to expose a relatively avascular area of the dura* (arrows).

incision begins approximately 2 mm posterior to the junction of the globe and optic nerve and continues for a length of 1.5 to 2 mm. This linear incision is then extended with long-handled transsphenoidal scissors for a total length of 3 to 5 mm (Fig 5).

A small Stevens tenotomy hook is then inserted into the subarachnoid space and moved anteriorly and posteriorly to lyse normal arachnoidal trabeculations and any adhesions that may develop with chronic distention of the dura. The hook is never moved too posteriorly to avoid damaging the central retinal artery, which traverses the subarachnoid space between 9 and 13 mm posterior to the junction of the optic nerve and globe.

We generally make three longitudinal incisions in the sheath rather than

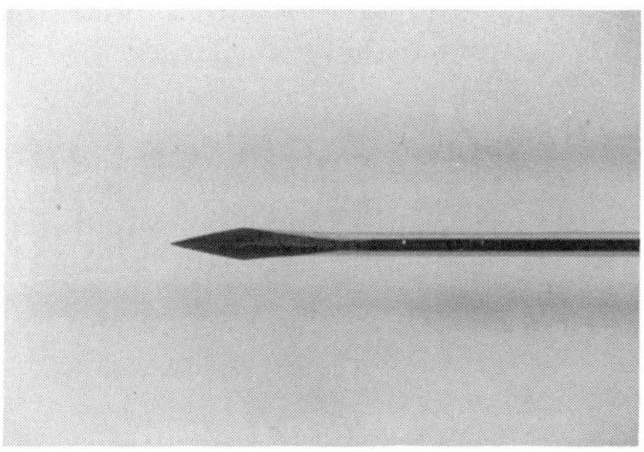

Figure 4 *Tympanic membrane blade used for incising the optic nerve meninges.*

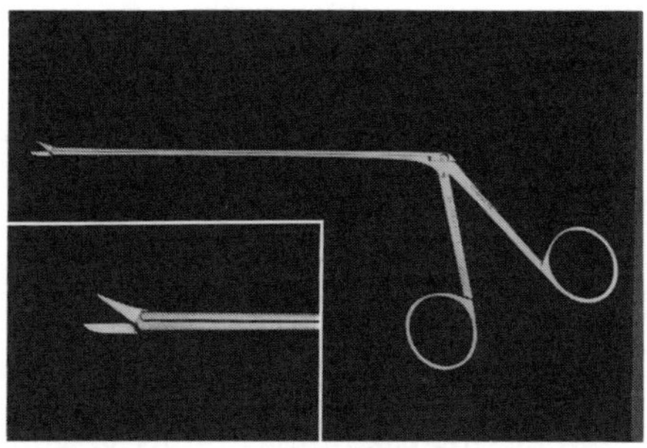

Figure 5 *Long-handled trans-sphenoidal scissors used to lengthen the initial dural incisions. High magnification (insert) illustrates the blunt tips. The nerve is not damaged when the lower immovable blade is inserted within the subarachnoid space.*

removing a rectangular dural window. No data exist, however, to recommend one technique in preference to the other. Occasionally, only two incisions can be made and, rarely, four can be placed. We do not believe that the number of incisions impacts directly on postoperative results. We never place just one incision, however, so that postoperative oozing of blood from the dura will not obstruct a single opening.

The traction sutures are removed, the medial rectus is reattached, and conjunctiva is closed with a running absorbable suture.

Lateral Approach

Tse and co-workers [10] described the lateral approach for ONSD. Although this technique has the advantage of exposing a longer segment of the nerve, considerably more surgery is required. Regardless of which approach is chosen, we do believe that operating microscope control of the optic nerve dissection is imperative. Failure to use the operating microscope (surgical loupes are not acceptable) entails too much risk of damage to the posterior ciliary arteries and ciliary nerves.

Postoperative Care

We maintain patients at absolute bed rest for the first 12 to 18 hours postoperatively. One to two hours after surgery, vision is checked as well as pupillary light reaction. Visual acuity is generally similar to the immediate preoperative status, although central vision may decrease by one to two lines of Snellen acuity.

Patients are examined for evidence of an orbital hemorrhage, and the posterior pole is examined with the direct ophthalmoscope to be certain that the central retinal artery is patent. Ice compresses are applied to the operated eye for 20 minutes every two hours for the first 12 to 18 hours.

On the morning of the first postoperative day, Snellen visual acuity is checked and patients are examined at the slit lamp. Ice compresses are continued every two hours while the patient is awake and erythromycin ophthalmic ointment is instilled into the inferior cul-de-sac twice daily and once before sleep. Unlimited ambulation except for lifting heavy objects and excessive bending over begins on the first postoperative day.

Patients remain hospitalized for 48 hours after the procedure and then are examined in one week. Subsequent follow-up examinations are scheduled according to each patient's progress.

Complications

The complications in our series of 200 optic nerve sheath decompressions has been reported recently [11]. The most disastrous complication is postoperative blindness. This irreversible complication has occurred in two patients and was due to central retinal artery occlusion. We have also had one patient lose vision permanently because of presumed traumatic optic neuropathy. It must be emphasized that patients should be fully appraised that ONSD may result in loss of sight.

Following the medial operative approach, the cornea adjacent to the limbus medially must be watched carefully for dellen formation. We have had one dellen develop an infection four weeks postoperatively, possibly related to the patient's use of constant nasal oxygen for chronic obstructive pulmonary disease.

Double vision, the most frequent complication, occurred in 9 of 200 patients. An adduction deficit developed within 72 hours of surgery in 8 patients. For 7, the diplopia was transient, resolving within one to four weeks. In one patient, permanent prismatic spectacle correction was required. The adduction deficit may be due to trauma to the medial rectus muscle or to its neural supply. In one other patient, a permanent 3-diopter esophoria also required prismatic correction.

One patient with a history of chronic dacryocystitis experienced a recurrence of this problem following ONSD. The dacryocystitis was treated with intravenous antibiotics with prompt resolution.

■ Indications

Pseudotumor Cerebri

Although pseudotumor cerebri (PTC) was once referred to as "benign intracranial hypertension," the careful retrospective study of Corbett and associates [12] demonstrated that PTC can result in significant loss of visual acuity and visual field in 50% of patients. Although lumboperitoneal shunts (LPSs) can effectively restore and preserve visual function, as mentioned earlier, cases of visual loss with functioning shunts have been well described and shunt complications are frequent.

ONSD, both by the medial and lateral approaches, has been shown to be effective for chronic papilledema associated with PTC [13–15]. The exact mechanism of visual improvement following ONSD is unknown, although relief of direct compression and vascular effects remains a possibility [16, 17]. Resolution of papilledema is prompt, usually beginning within the first 48 hours after surgery.

Surgery in one eye will often benefit the other eye. This contralateral effect has been hypothesized to be due to filtration of cerebrospinal fluid through the posterior orbit and chiasm [16]. Seif and Shah [17] demonstrated with a biomechanical model that such a mechanism has validity.

Relief of headache due to increased intracranial pressure following ONSD is variable. If a patient's primary problem is headache, then an LPS should be performed. Patients with both headache and visual loss may eventually require both surgical procedures to manage their problems.

Chronic Papilledema Due to Nonresectable Central Nervous System Mass

Some mass lesions are unable to be resected from the venous drainage system of the brain. We have seen this syndrome with arteriovenous malformation of the vein of Galen, meningiomas of the falx, and prostate carcinoma metastatic to the region of the superior sagittal sinus.

Chronic papilledema develops in these patients, which ultimately produces severely contracted visual fields and loss of visual acuity. ONSD should be performed early in the course of these patients' illness. These patients usually are referred for evaluation after profound visual loss has occurred. Optic nerve surgery will halt the progression of visual deficits, but this surgical intervention has not restored vision for these patients. Treatment with diuretics and corticosteroids has only temporary effects and has not been satisfactory.

Postdecompression Blindness

Postdecompression blindness is a rare syndrome in which visual loss develops after successful removal of the tumor in patients with central nervous system mass lesions and papilledema [18, 19]. Scarring of the subarachnoid space at the posterior orbital apex presumably traps cerebrospinal fluid under high pressure within the intraorbital optic nerve.

Visual loss usually occurs three to six weeks after neurosurgical resection of the mass lesion, but we have seen cases evolve at earlier and later times in the postoperative course. This syndrome is a purely mechanical closed space, "compartment" syndrome and must be treated aggressively with ONSD. As in the situation of nonresectable central nervous system mass lesions, medical management is of no value.

Following neurosurgery, patients must be monitored for ophthalmoscopic signs that the chronic papilledema is resolving. If patients have severe visual loss at the time of diagnosis of the central nervous system mass lesion, there may be a role for simultaneous decompression of the optic nerves and resection of the tumor.

Postoperative Subarachnoid Hemorrhage of Optic Nerve

On rare occasions, the needle used for retrobulbar anesthetic injections for intraocular surgery may produce a subarachnoid hemorrhage of the optic nerve [20]. Any patient in whom a central retinal vein occlusion (CRVO) or combined central retinal artery occlusion (CRAO) and CRVO develop within 24 hours to seven days postoperatively has blood in the subarachnoid space. A-scan and B-scan ultrasonography as well as CT and magnetic resonance imaging may not demonstrate the subarachnoid blood and may not reveal enlargement of the optic nerve meningeal complex. ONSD should not be delayed because of normal imaging studies, however, because a significant amount of blood may accumulate within the subarachnoid space and yet be below the resolution capability of these imaging systems.

The visual prognosis in these patients appears to be related to the degree of retinal ischemia present at the time of surgery. When ONSD is performed, the cataract incision must be reinforced with additional sutures to prevent prolapse of the intraocular contents during traction on the globe.

Acute Retinal Necrosis Syndrome

Because some patients with acute retinal necrosis (ARN) syndrome have visual loss primarily caused by an optic neuropathy [21], ONSD has been performed for these patients with some encouraging visual results [22]. Because ONSD appears to improve the flow of blood through the central retinal artery as judged by color Doppler imaging [23], this procedure may also benefit perfusion of the posterior pole and peripheral retina.

Nonarteritic Ischemic Optic Neuropathy

The use of ONSD for the progressive form of nonarteritic ischemic optic neuropathy (NAION) is highly controversial [24]. Sergott and colleagues [24] reported significant visual improvement for 12 of 14 patients undergoing ONSD for this disorder compared with permanent visual loss in the unoperated control group.

As anticipated, this article sparked a great deal of debate [25]. These findings, however, have now been reproduced at other centers [8]. In addition, studies using color Doppler study indicate that ONSD improves systolic velocity of blood flow through the ophthalmic artery and decreases the vascular resistance of the posterior ciliary system in patients with NAION [26]. Therefore, hemodynamic changes may explain the phenomenon of visual improvement following ONSD for ischemia of the optic nerve.

Central Retinal Vein Occlusion

Although reports from South America have reported visual improvement following ONSD for CRVO, these studies are poorly documented and do not offer precise clinical details [27, 28].

The combined experience of Wills Eye Hospital and the University of Utah (Richard Anderson, M.D.) has not demonstrated significant visual improvement for patients with CRVO present for six months or longer. Whether ONSD has any role for more acute CRVOs will require a long-term and complex prospective, randomized clinical trial.

■ Summary

Despite skepticism regarding the efficacy of the procedure, ONSD now has an established role in the management of visual loss associated with chronic papilledema. The surgical procedure requires microscopic dissection of the intraorbital optic nerve to avoid permanent damage to the nerve and its vascular supply. Recent (albeit controversial) investigations concerning ONSD for ischemic disease of the optic nerve suggest that the procedure may have more pathophysiological effects than were once believed.

■ References

1. DeWecker L. An incision of the optic nerve in cases of neuroretinitis. First Ophthalmol Congress Report 1872;4:11–14
2. Carter RB. Case of swollen optic disc in which the sheath of the optic nerve was incised behind the eyeball. Proc Med Soc (London) 1887;20:290

3. Hayreh SS. Pathogenesis of oedema of the optic disc. Doc Ophthalmol 1968; 24:289–411
4. Davidson SI. A surgical approach to plerocephalic disc. Doc Ophthalmol 1969; 89:669–690
5. Galbraith JEK, Sullivan JH. Decompression of the perioptic meninges for relief of papilledema. Am J Ophthalmol 1973;73:687–692
6. Kilpatrick CJ, Kaufman DV, Galbraith JEK, et al. Optic nerve decompression in benign intracranial hypertension. Clin Exp Neurol 1981;18:161–168
7. Rosenberg M, Smith C, Beck R, et al. The efficacy of shunting procedures in pseudotumor cerebri. Neurology 1989;39:209
8. Kelman SE, Sergott RC, Cioffi GA, et al. Modified optic nerve decompression in patients with functioning lumboperitoneal shunts and progressive visual loss. Ophthalmology 1991 (in press)
9. Sergott RC. Diagnosis and management of vision threatening papilledema. Semin Neurol 1986;6:176–184
10. Tse DT, Nerad JA, Anderson RL, Corbett JJ. Optic nerve sheath fenestration in pseudotumor cerebri. A lateral orbitotomy approach. Arch Ophthalmol 1988;106: 1458–1462
11. Sergott RC, Savino PJ, Bosley TM. Optic nerve decompression: a clinical review and proposed pathophysiologic mechanism. Aust NZ J Ophthalmol 1990;18:365–373
12. Corbett JJ, Savino PJ, Thompson HS, et al. Visual loss in pseudotumor cerebri. Arch Neurol 1982;38:461–474
13. Brourman ND, Spoor TC, Ramocki JM. Optic nerve sheath decompression for pseudotumor cerebri. Arch Ophthalmol 1988;106:1378–1383
14. Sergott RC, Savino PJ, Bosley TM. Modified optic nerve decompression provides long-term visual improvement in pseudotumor cerebri. Arch Ophthalmol 1988; 106:1384–1390
15. Corbett JJ, Nerad JA, Tse DT, Anderson RL. Results of optic nerve sheath fenestration for pseudotumor cerebri: the lateral orbitotomy approach. Arch Ophthalmol 1988;106:1391–1397
16. Keltner JL. Editorial: optic nerve sheath decompression: how does it work? Has its time come? Arch Ophthalmol 1988;106:1365–1369
17. Seif SL, Shah L. A model for the mechanism of optic nerve sheath fenestration. Arch Ophthalmol 1990;108:1326–1329
18. Beck RW, Greenberg HS. Post-decompression optic neuropathy. J Neurosurg 1985;63:196–199
19. Saul RF, Thurston SE, Sergott RC. Visual loss following craniotomy for obstructive hydrocephalus. Presented at the Frank Walsh Society, Salt Lake City, UT, February 1991
20. Sullivan KL, Brown GC, Forman AR, et al. Retrobulbar anesthesia and retinal vascular obstruction. Ophthalmology 1983;90:373–377
21. Sergott RC, Belmont JB, Savino PJ, et al. Optic nerve involvement in the acute retinal necrosis syndrome. Arch Ophthalmol 1985;103:1160–1162
22. Sergott RC, Anand R, Belmont JB, et al. Acute retinal necrosis neuropathy: clinical profile and surgical therapy. Arch Ophthalmol 1989;107:692–696
23. Flaharty P, Leib W, Sergott RC, et al. Optic nerve sheath decompression improves blood flow to the retinal circulation. Presented at VIII International Neuro-Ophthalmology Symposium, Winchester, England, June 1990
24. Sergott RC, Cohen MS, Bosley TM, Savino PJ. Optic nerve decompression may improve the progressive form of nonarteritic ischemic optic neuropathy. Arch Ophthalmol 1989;107:1743–1754
25. Letter to Editor. Arch Ophthalmol 1990;108:1063–1068
26. Flaharty P, Leib W, Sergott RC, et al. ONSO improves blood flow velocity and

decreases vascular resistance in ischemic optic neuropathy. Presented at the 17th North American Neuro-ophthalmology Society, Park City, Utah, February 1991

27. Vasco-Posada J. Modification of the circulation in the posterior pole of the eye. Ann Ophthalmol 1972;10:48–59
28. Arcinieqas A. Treatment of the occlusion of the central retinal vein by section of the posterior ring. Ann Ophthalmol 1984;16:1081–1086

Retinal and Optic Nerve Head Disorders Masquerading as Diseases of the Central Nervous System

J. Donald M. Gass, M.D.
Saunders L. Hupp, M.D.

Visual loss from primary disease of the retina and anterior optic nerve may masquerade as central nervous system disease due to a common ophthalmoscopic appearance. Affected patients often present with one or a combination of three unexplained findings: (1) elevation and enlargement of the optic nerve head, (2) visual loss without fundus changes, and (3) optic atrophy. A thorough history and eye examination combined with selection of a few ancillary studies in all but a few cases will permit ophthalmologists to make the correct diagnosis and avoid unnecessary neurological investigations.

■ Pseudopapilledema

The term *papilledema* will be confined to blurring of the optic disc margins and swelling of the optic nerve head caused by increased intracranial pressure, and the term *pseudopapilledema* will be used to describe all of the causes of disc changes that may appear identical to or be mistaken for papilledema.

Fluorescein angiography and ultrasonography may be helpful in differentiating papilledema from some causes of pseudopapilledema. Angiography in all stages of papilledema typically shows dilation and permeability alterations of juxtapapillary retinal capillaries that extend beyond the edge of the optic disc swelling. The appearance time of the dye and retinal circulation time are usually not altered except in some cases of severe papilledema. Dynamic echographic evaluation using the 30-degree test [1] is helpful in detecting expansion of the optic nerve sheaths by subarachnoid fluid in patients with increased intracranial pressure. Although this finding is present in virtually all patients with increased intracranial pressure and papilledema, it may also occur with other disorders affecting the anterior part of the optic nerve [2, 3].

Congenital Anomalies

Hyperopia Relatively small eyes of some patients may have elevation of the optic nerve head by virtue of having a near normal number of nerve

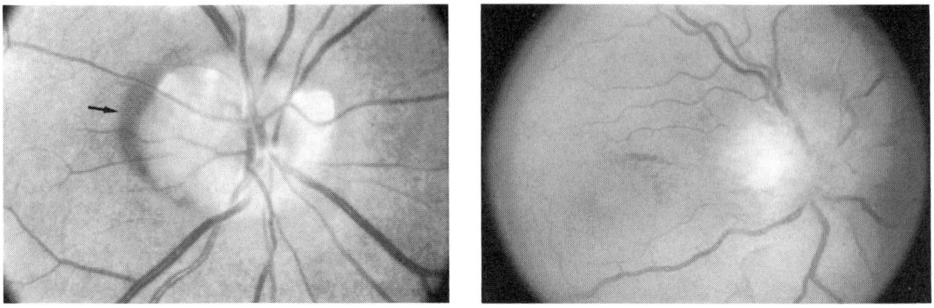

A B

Figure 1 *Drusen of optic disc. (A) Calcified drusen and rim of subretinal blood* (arrow). *(B) Acute optic neuropathy. Drusen became apparent as disc swelling disappeared and acuity returned to normal. (From [4]. Used with permission.)*

fibers traversing a small optic canal. Visual function is normal, and cycloplegic refraction is all that is usually necessary to differentiate these prominent optic discs with small or no cups from papilledema. Ultrasound to demonstrate a small eye and absence of expansion of the optic nerve sheaths, as well as fluorescein angiography to demonstrate absence of capillary dilation extending beyond the optic disc margins, are other studies that may be used if the diagnosis is uncertain.

Drusen of the Optic Disc These nodular deposits of extracellular material that are located anterior to the lamina cribrosa within the optic nerve head may be present at birth or may develop following birth. In infancy and childhood these deposits, which are sometimes referred to as hyaline bodies, may cause diffuse swelling of the optic nerve head yet may not be visible ophthalmoscopically. Only later in life do the drusen become obvious as they become more calcified [4] (Fig 1A). This material may crowd the surrounding nerve fibers and produce variable degrees of compression atrophy, elevation of the nerve head, lateral displacement of the surrounding retina, and occasionally juxtapapillary subretinal neovascularization. Visual loss may occur abruptly because of hemorrhage or exudation from juxtapapillary subretinal neovascularization or because of acute swelling of the nerve head, presumably by vascular obstruction (Fig 1B). In some cases there may be return of normal function whereas in others optic atrophy and permanent loss of vision may occur. Gradual loss of visual field, particularly nasally with optic atrophy, may be caused by progressive accumulation of drusen in the nerve head.

Angiography shows minimal evidence of retinal capillary dilation beyond the area of disc swelling, but it does reveal late staining of the nerve head. Ultrasound and computed tomography can detect calcified drusen, but, particularly in young children with less calcified drusen, these tests may not be helpful in the differential diagnosis. Because drusen may be inherited as an autosomal dominant pattern, examination of other family members is helpful.

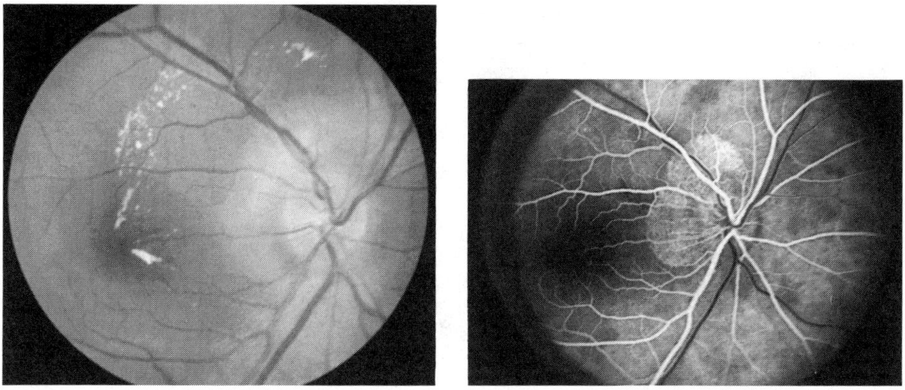

A B

Figure 2 *Juxtapapillary capillary hemangioma. (A) Juxtapapillary angioma misdiagnosed as papilledema in woman complaining of headaches. (B) Early angiogram showing capillary angioma. (From [5]. Copyright © 1974 by the American Medical Association. Used with permission.)*

Sessile Capillary Hemangiomas (von Hippel's Disease) Slightly elevated capillary hemangiomas arising within the juxtapapillary retina and optic nerve head may cause a picture simulating papilledema [5] (Fig 2). These hamartomas often occur unilaterally but may be bilateral and occasionally may be associated with peripheral retinal angiomas. In approximately 10% of patients, angiomas may involve the cerebellum and spinal cord. Visual loss is caused by intraretinal and subretinal exudation that is usually associated with yellowish lipid exudates surrounding the area of exudation.

Biomicroscopy and stereoscopic early-phase fluorescein angiography is important in differentiating this lesion from papilledema, juxtapapillary subretinal neovascularization, or a juxtapapillary choroidal hemangioma [5]. Stereoangiographically, capillary angiomas show superficial optic nerve and retinal vessels extending downward into the area of the capillary angioma. Early in their development, these angiomas may be difficult to detect ophthalmoscopically and may be misinterpreted angiographically as focal areas of optic neuritis. The growth rate of these lesions is variable. Treatment with argon green laser may be of benefit in reducing exudation but must be done with care to avoid excessive damage either to the optic nerve or the nerve fiber layer.

Combined Retinal and Pigment Epithelial Hamartomas These lesions are composed of a capillary angiomatous and a pigment epithelial component (Fig 3). When the former outweighs the latter, they may appear quite similar to sessile capillary angiomas. Angiographically, their capillary component is quite evident. They cause visual loss primarily by contraction of the vitreoretinal interface over the tumor, producing retinal folds extending into the macula and less frequently by exudation. A small percentage of these patients will show manifestations of neurofibromatosis [6].

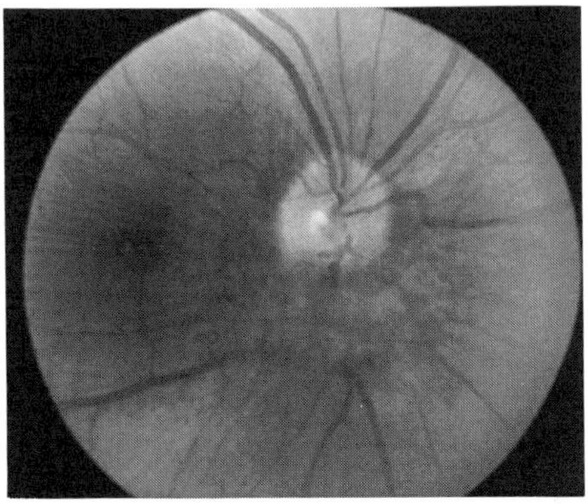

Figure 3 *Combined retinal and pigment epithelial hamartoma. Typical lesion with pigmentation and retinal folds extending into macula. Patient had neurilemoma excised from ipsilateral orbit.*

Leber's Hereditary Optic Neuropathy This disorder affects predominantly young adult men and typically begins with acute or subacute loss of central vision in one eye followed soon afterward in the second eye. Circumpapillary telangiectatic microangiopathy, swelling of the nerve fiber layer around the optic disc, and absence of staining on fluorescein angiography are characteristic of this disorder (Fig 4). Many asymptomatic family members with the disease have peripapillary microangiopathy. The telangiectatic changes disappear as atrophy of the optic nerve develops. The primary locus of the disease appears to be the intraocular rather than the retrobulbar area, and Leber's hereditary vascular neuroretinopathy may be a more appropriate name. Dilation of the optic nerve sheath may be present at the time of acute visual loss and may prove to be of importance in the pathogenesis of acute visual loss. Mitochondrial DNA mutation has been identified in affected members [7].

Other Congenital Anomalies of the Disc A variety of anomalies of the optic disc may be misinterpreted as papilledema, particularly in patients with visual complaints in the affected eye.

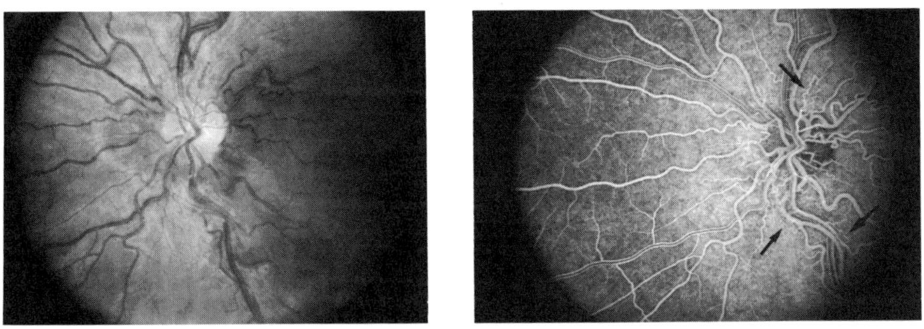

A B

Figure 4 *(A, B) Leber's optic neuropathy in 18-year-old man with 2-week history of blurred vision. Angiography shows telangiectatic vessels* (arrows). *(From [4]. Used with permission.)*

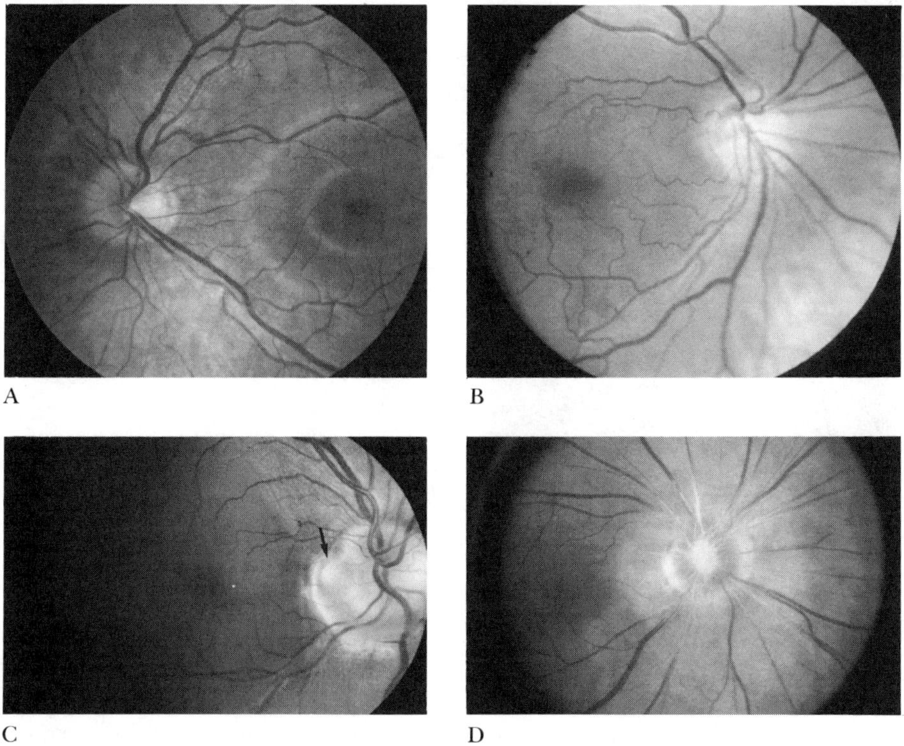

Figure 5 *Anomalies of optic disc mistaken for papilledema. (A, B) Tilted optic disc. (C) Congenital pit* (arrow) *of optic disc (white dot artifact). (D) "Morning glory" deformity.*

Marked tilting of the optic disc may be associated with segmental elevation of the margin of the optic disc, usually on the side away from the tilt (Fig 5A). In most cases, patients are asymptomatic and have normal visual function. In some cases, however, particularly with severe tilting of the disc in an inferotemporal direction, there may be a superior visual field defect related to anomalous development of the retina and optic nerve (Fig 5B).

Congenital pit of the optic nerve is always associated with some enlargement of the diameter of the optic disc and causes visual loss by virtue of serous exudation into the subretinal space. This latter detachment may be shallow and relatively inapparent. The optic pit is usually present near the temporal margin of the optic disc and often appears as a dark round depression (Fig 5C). Some patients with optic pits have a centrocecal visual field defect even in the presence of normal acuity and in the absence of any evidence of retinal detachment.

When viewed monocularly, enlarged colobomatous optic discs may be misinterpreted as being elevated rather than depressed. Likewise, mild juxtapapillary staphylomas may be associated with a slight change in the color of the pigment epithelium and may be mistaken for elevation of the disc margin, when in fact it is due to a depression in the tissue surrounding the optic disc.

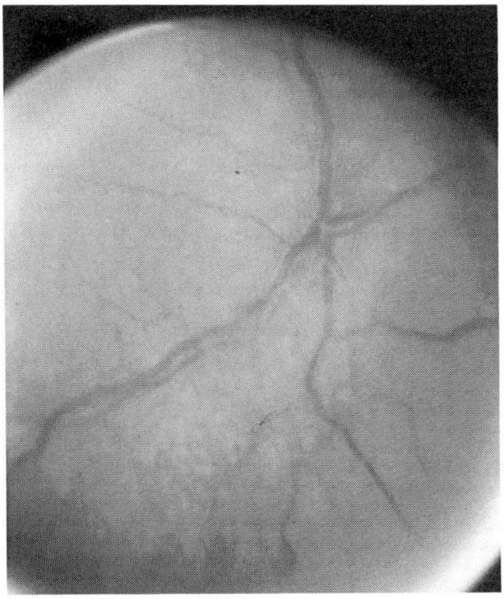

Figure 6 *Pseudopapilledema in 19-month-old boy with Leber's amaurosis. (From [8]. Used with permission.)*

Some of these patients are subject to transient loss of central vision that may be caused by episodic contraction of anomalous presence of smooth muscle within the anterior optic nerve sheath. Visible contractions of the juxtapapillary tissue around the optic nerve may occasionally be seen. When the center portion of the colobomatous depression in the nerve head is filled with glial tissue, its appearance has been referred to as the "morning glory" deformity (Fig 5D).

Leber's Congenital Amaurosis Leber's congenital amaurosis is an infantile tapetoretinal dystrophy that is characterized by blindness or very low vision at birth, failure to fix, nystagmus, and sluggish pupils. Although many of these infants are otherwise normal, probably half or more will exhibit other neurological signs. The ocular fundi at birth may appear normal, but mild swelling and pallor of the optic disc may be present and may be confused with papilledema [8] (Fig 6). The electroretinogram, which is extinguished in most patients and markedly abnormal in the remainder, is essential in differentiating this disorder from other causes of congenital blindness.

Inflammatory Disorders (Papillitis)

Acute Postviral Neuroretinitis (Leber's Idiopathic Stellate Neuroretinopathy) This syndrome is characterized by acute unilateral loss of vision, swelling of the optic nerve head, and juxtapapillary exudative retinal detachment, usually in patients recovering from a viral-like illness (Fig 7). A macular star more prominent on the nasal side of the fovea usually appears within several days and becomes more prominent as the disc elevation subsides. One or more focal white areas of retinitis may be present in approximately 10% of cases [9]. Vitreous cells are present in approximately 90% of patients. The visual function and the appearance of the fundus usually return to normal

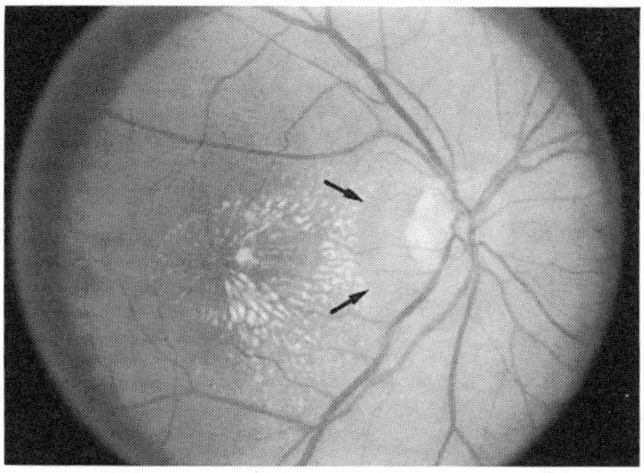

Figure 7 *Leber's stellate neuroretinopathy in a woman with acute loss of vision in the right eye following a flu-like syndrome.* Arrows *indicate juxtapapillary exudative retinal detachment.*

within three to six months without treatment. A few patients may be left with mild pallor of the optic disc.

Angiography shows staining of the optic disc that persists for weeks after disappearance of optic disc swelling. The macular star may persist for many weeks or months. Focal areas of leakage are demonstrated in the disc of the opposite eye in 5 to 10% of patients.

Diffuse Unilateral Subacute Neuroretinitis Diffuse unilateral subacute neuroretinitis (DUSN) is a clinical syndrome characterized by acute visual loss, vitritis, papillitis, retinal vasculitis, and recurrent crops of evanescent gray/white outer retinal lesions and later by progressive visual loss, optic atrophy, retinal vessel narrowing, and diffuse, as well as multifocal, areas of retinal pigment epithelium degeneration [10]. It is caused by an as yet unidentified nematode that may wander within the subretinal space and cause progressive ocular damage.

A variety of ophthalmoscopic pictures may be present. In some, the fundus may appear essentially normal. In most there is mild disc swelling. A single cluster of small white lesions at the level of the pigment epithelium may or may not be present (Fig 8A). These focal areas of retinitis are caused by material left in the subretinal space by the nematode, which can usually be located biomicroscopically in the area of these exudates. Early, the visual acuity may be mildly or severely affected. A Marcus Gunn pupillary reaction is usually present. The white lesions fade within a matter of a few days. In some patients extensive perivascular exudation simulating that seen in sarcoidosis may occur. Thiabendazole and diethylcarbamazine are usually ineffective in destroying the nematode unless a severe vitreous inflammatory reaction is present. Successful treatment usually requires biomicroscopic identification of the nematode and its destruction with photocoagulation. Failure to find the nematode leads to progressive optic atrophy and narrowing of the retinal vessels and pigmentary generation throughout the affected eye (Fig 8B).

Sarcoidosis Granulomatous infiltration of the optic nerve head in sarcoidosis may simulate papilledema and may be associated with visual loss. In most instances some nodularity of the optic disc swelling is evident and is a clue to the presence of granulomas (Fig 9) [4]. Ophthalmoscopic and angiographic evidence of retinal periphlebitis may be present (see Fig 9B). Patients with

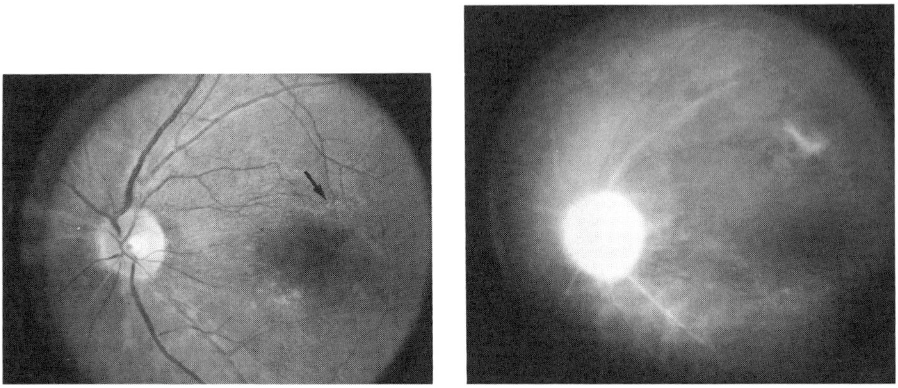

A B

Figure 8 *Diffuse unilateral subacute neuroretinitis. (A) Acute visual loss in this boy was misdiagnosed as optic neuritis. Note small foci of outer retinitis and nematode* (arrow) *that was unrecognized. (B) Several years later. Note severe optic atrophy and retinal vessel narrowing.*

optic nerve head involvement are likely to have involvement of the central nervous system.

Aphakic Cystoid Macular Edema Aphakic cystoid macular edema is a common cause of loss of central vision in patients after cataract extraction. It is often associated with very mild evidence of optic disc edema, but in some cases the edema may be severe (Fig 10). Biomicroscopic and angiographic demonstration of cysts in the macular is important in differentiating the disc swelling from that caused by increased intracranial pressure.

Chronic Vitritis Optic disc edema or cystoid macular edema may develop in patients with bilateral chronic vitritis. These patients can be subdivided

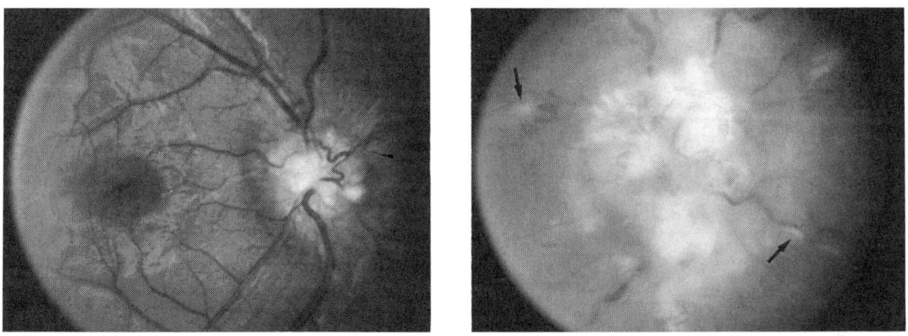

A B

Figure 9 *Sarcoid papillitis. (A, B) Note nodular aspect of swelling caused by granulomas and perivenous exudation* (arrows). *(A from [4]. Used with permission.)*

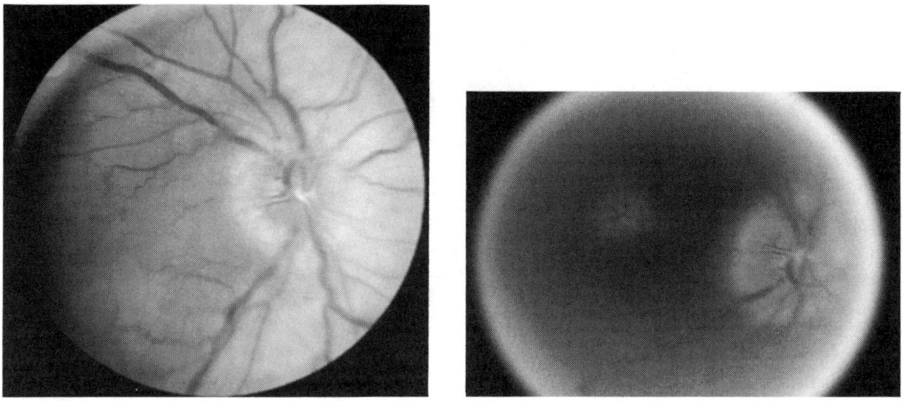

A B

Figure 10 *Aphakic cystoid macular edema and optic disc edema. (A) Optic disc swelling. (B) Late phase angiogram with cystoid macular edema.*

into at least three categories based on the associated findings. (1) Pars planitis with vitreous inflammation associated with snowbank exudate overlying the peripheral retina and pars plana, usually in the inferior fundus of both eyes. This disorder most commonly occurs in children and young adults who are otherwise in excellent health. Snowball opacities in the inferior vitreous similar to those seen in sarcoidosis are often present. (2) Senile vitritis occurs usually in patients 50 years of age or older and may be associated with some irregular changes in the retinal pigment epithelium in the equatorial portion of the fundus [11]. It is more common in women than in men. (3) Vitiliginous, or birdshot, chorioretinitis also affects predominantly middle aged and older women and is associated with the development of multiple ill-defined areas of yellowish depigmentation of the uveal melanocytes that are most prominent in the postequatorial region surrounding the nasal two-thirds of the optic disc [12]. Progressive narrowing of the retinal vessels and pallor of the optic disc slowly develop in these patients and is associated with clinical as well as electrophysiological evidence of rod and cone dysfunction.

The Presumed Ocular Histoplasmosis Syndrome Presumed ocular histoplasmosis syndrome (POHS), which is endemic in the eastern half of the United States, is characterized by the presence of multifocal areas of chorioretinal and juxtapapillary scarring. These scars may enlarge and in some cases be associated with a localized transient exudative retinal detachment presumably caused by recurrent lymphocytic infiltration. Occasionally a patient will present with a temporal scotoma associated with juxtapapillary exudative detachment of the retina that may be misdiagnosed as papilledema. The exudation disappears spontaneously and leaves patients with a juxtapapillary atrophic pigment epithelial scar. It is important to differentiate this cause of juxtapapillary detachment from that caused more frequently by subretinal neovascularization arising from a preexisting juxtapapillary scar in patients with POHS.

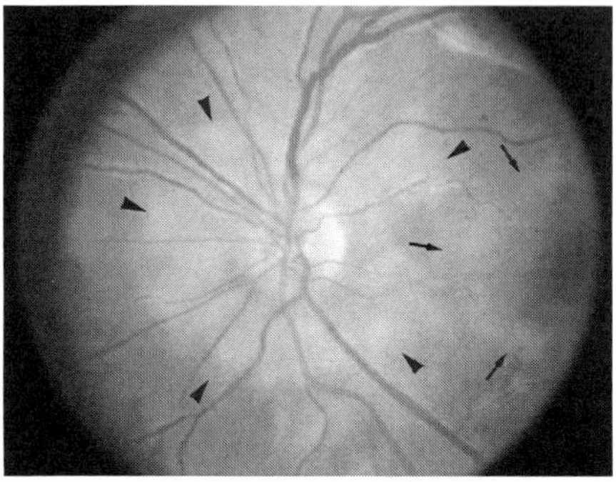

Figure 11 *Pseudopapilledema caused by acute posterior multifocal placoid pigment epitheliopathy with bilateral juxtapapillary* (arrowheads) *and macular* (arrows) *placoid lesions. (From [4]. Used with permission.)*

Pseudo-POHS Syndrome (Multifocal Choroiditis and Panuveitis) These patients may present with visual loss associated with multifocal areas of active choroiditis and juxtapapillary choroiditis, which is usually associated with evidence of inactive chorioretinal scars identical to that seen in POHS [13]. Vitreous inflammatory cells are usually present. There is accumulating evidence that this syndrome may occasionally occur in association with the multiple evanescent white dot syndrome and the acute idiopathic blind spot enlargement syndrome (see discussion below).

Acute Posterior Multifocal Placoid Pigment Epitheliopathy and Serpiginous Choroiditis Occasionally a patient with these disorders may present with symptoms related to acute gray white lesions at the level of the pigment epithelium confined to the area surrounding the optic disc, which may be mistaken for papilledema (Fig 11) [4]. Fluorescein angiography is helpful in such cases in making the correct diagnosis.

Acute Occult Outer Zonal Retinitis (Multiple Evanescent White Dot Syndrome) and Acute Idiopathic Blind Spot Enlargement Syndrome Multiple evanescent white dot syndrome was first described in 1984 as a new self-limited inflammatory disorder primarily causing visual loss and electroretinographic changes in one eye of young women with multiple evanescent white lesions affecting the outer retina [14]. Photopsias, temporal scotoma, and characteristic fluorescein angiographic changes were later emphasized (Fig 12). In 1988, acute idiopathic blind spot enlargement syndrome was described in young women, usually in one eye associated with no fundus changes but with electroretinographic abnormalities [15]. It is probable that these two syndromes are part of the protean manifestation of the same disease that causes acute damage to the retinal photoreceptor elements in one or more large zones of the ocular fundus, usually including the juxtapapillary area, less frequently the macular area, and often a large sector of the peripheral fundus. Prominent and dense enlargement of the blind spot is a frequent feature of the disease but is not present in all cases. Swelling of the optic disc occurs occasionally and incorrectly suggests that visual loss is primarily caused by optic neuritis. This diagnosis should be suspected in any patient (even a man) presenting with acute visual loss associated with photopsias and a temporal scotoma in one eye. Those patients who demonstrate multiple small ill-defined round spots at the level

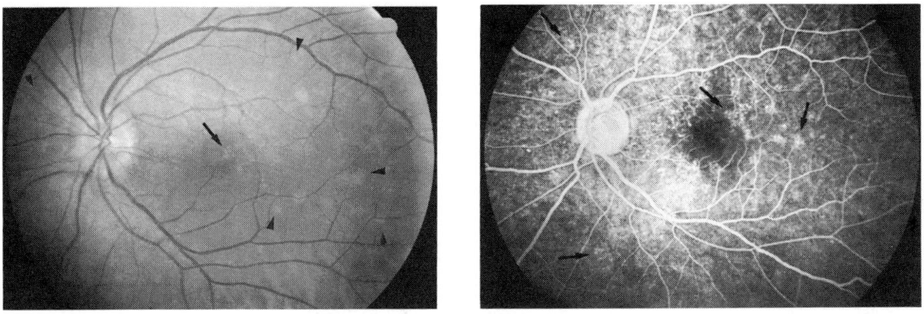

A B

Figure 12 *Multiple evanescent white dot syndrome in young woman with acute onset visual loss, photopsia, and enlarged blind spot in the left eye. (A)* Arrow *indicates cluster of orange foveal dots, and* arrowheads *indicate the white outer retinal lesions. (B) Early phase angiogram shows clusters of hyperfluorescent dots* (arrows).

of the pigment epithelium will show a characteristic fluorescein angiographic finding of a wreath-like pattern of punctate hyperfluorescence and late staining, as well as staining of the optic disc (see Fig 12). In those patients who show no evidence of abnormality in the fundus, the finding of abnormal electroretinographic changes is important in arriving at the correct diagnosis [15]. Although initial reports suggested that spontaneous recovery occurs within several months, there is now evidence that permanent visual field changes and prolonged complaints of photopsia may result.

Occlusive Vascular Papillopathy

Malignant Hypertension Patients with undiagnosed accelerated hypertension may present with reduced visual acuity or transient obscurations of vision and show evidence of optic disc swelling in one or both eyes. Hemorrhages or exudates that suggest severe hypertension may not always be obvious [4]. The presence of a macular star figure may lead to a misdiagnosis of Leber's stellate neuroretinitis (Fig 13). Focal narrowing of the retinal arteries in these cases is usually a clue to the nature of the swollen optic disc.

Anterior Ischemic Optic Neuropathy Patients with anterior ischemic optic neuropathy (AION), particularly those with nonarteritic AION, typically present with acute altitudinal visual field loss and show swelling of the optic disc that may be diffuse or segmental. One or more flame-shaped hemorrhages are often present. Fluorescein angiography often shows some delay in retinal artery appearance time, increase in retinal circulation time, and staining of the optic disc. In arteritic AION the swollen optic nerve head often appears remarkably pale.

Acute Disc Swelling in Juvenile Diabetes Patients with long-standing juvenile diabetes may develop mild blurring of vision in one or both eyes associated with disc swelling, presumably related to a reversible vasculopathy, because most show clearing of the edema and return of normal vision without specific therapy [16].

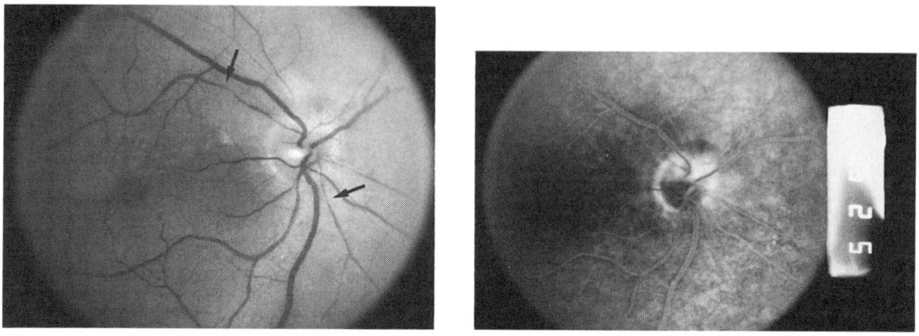

A B

Figure 13 *Disc edema and macular star misdiagnosed as Leber's stellate neuroretinopathy in a patient with undiagnosed hypertension and blood pressure of 260/140. (A) Note focal narrowing of retinal arterioles* (arrows). *(B) Segmental staining of the optic disc as seen on fluorescein angiography. (From [4]. Used with permission.)*

Venous Stasis Papillopathy (Papillophlebitis) These patients are typically young or middle-age adults who present with mild blurring of vision in one eye associated with swelling of the optic nerve head, mild venous engorgement, and a few retinal hemorrhages that are largely limited to the area surrounding the optic disc [17]. Visual field examination is characterized by an enlarged blind spot. Most patients experience spontaneous recovery without any treatment, and the fundus usually returns to normal.

Neoplastic Papillopathy

Patients may present with swelling of the optic nerve head, usually in one eye, caused by a neoplasm in the retrobulbar area or by direct invasion of the nerve head (Fig 14).

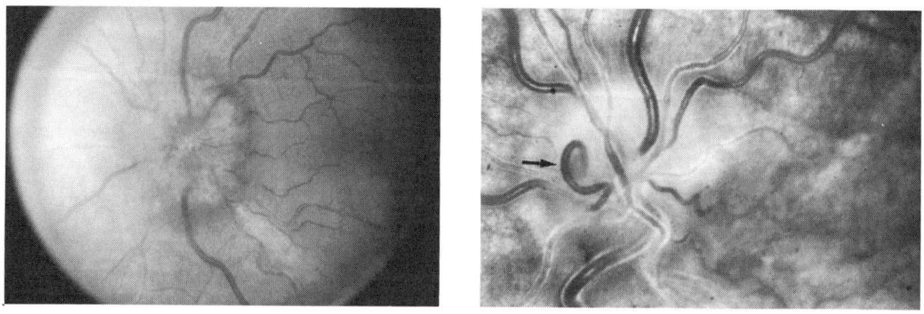

A B

Figure 14 *Meningioma of the optic nerve. (A) Diffuse disc edema is evident in July 1977. (B) Several years later. Note optic atrophy and venous collaterals* (arrow).

Optic Disc-Vitreous Interface Contraction and Traction

Spontaneous contraction of a fibrocellular membrane on the optic disc surface may cause sudden blurring of vision and a fundus picture simulating papilledema. This condition is usually unilateral but may be bilateral, particularly in patients with chronic vitritis. Extensive posterior vitreous detachment with remaining attachments in the juxtapapillary area may create vitreous traction and produce swelling of the optic disc [4].

■ "Normal" Fundus and Visual Loss

Cone Dystrophy or Progressive Cone Degeneration

This genetically determined condition may begin at any age, and in its early stages it may be unassociated with any ophthalmoscopic changes. Most cases are sporadic, but when they are familial most are autosomal dominant. Clinical symptoms include progressive loss of central vision, impairment of color vision, photophobia, and hemeralopia. Visual acuity varies from 20/20 early, to 20/200 or less later. Although the fundus may be initially normal, depigmentation of the pigment epithelium, often in a bull's-eye pattern, usually begins within several years of onset of symptoms. In a few patients, temporal pallor of the optic disc may be the only fundus change. Some patients may later develop evidence of rod dysfunction. Electroretinography is essential in establishing the diagnosis of cone dystrophy. Cone dystrophy is one of the most common disorders masquerading as a central nervous system disease. Many patients may not complain of photophobia and loss of color vision. In the early stages, the extent of cone degeneration may be inadequate to detect using standard electroretinography.

Stargardt's Disease (Fundus Flavimaculatus)

Stargardt's disease is usually inherited as an autosomal recessive disorder, that is characterized by the onset of loss of central vision during childhood, early adulthood, or occasionally, middle age. Initially, there may be only a vermillion color to the fundus. Later, evidence of yellowish flecks often confined to the paracentral region appear, and are accompanied by a bull's eye or oval pattern of pigment epithelial atrophy. These flecks are variable in size, shape, and distribution (Fig 15).

Stargardt's disease is a lipofuscin storage disorder affecting the retinal pigment epithelium and it is the thickening of the pigment epithelium by this lipofuscin that is responsible for the vermillion color to the fundus and for the characteristic angiographic findings of obscuration of the choroidal fluorescence, except in those areas of pigment epithelial atrophy.

Sex-linked Juvenile Retinoschisis

Patients with sex-linked juvenile retinoschisis typically present in their early school years because of reading difficulty. Although the fundus may appear normal on ophthalmoscopic examination, biomicroscopic examination

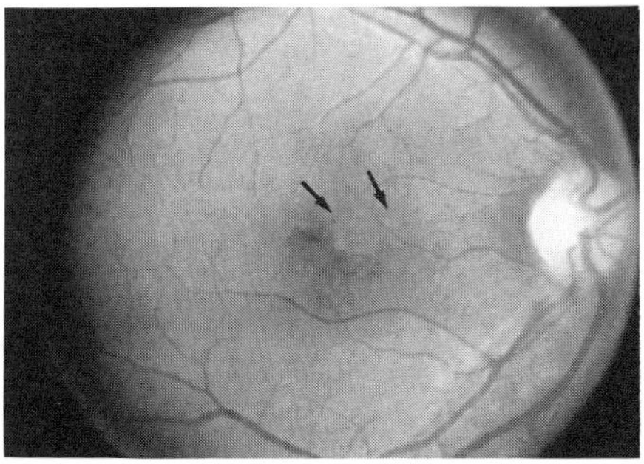

A

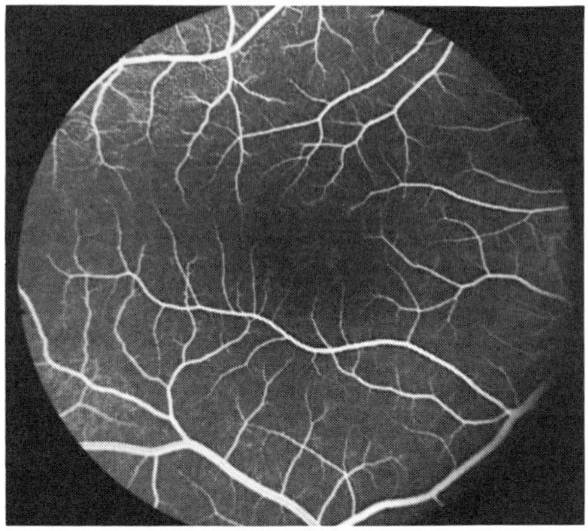

B

Figure 15 *Stargardt's disease. (A) The fundus was interpreted as normal, but note areas of retinal pigment epithelial atrophy* (arrows). *(B) The angiogram shows dark choroid and faint fluorescence centrally corresponding to areas of pigment atrophy.*

reveals characteristic superficially located small cysts arranged in a stellate pattern and radial striae centered in the foveal area of both eyes present from birth (Fig 16). Fifty percent of patients will have evidence of peripheral retinoschisis. Visual acuity is usually in the range of 20/40 to 20/200. Only men are affected, and there are no ocular changes present in the carriers. Fluorescein angiography is normal in 50% of cases and shows mottled hyperfluorescence in the remainder of cases. Electroretinography usually reveals abnormalities that primarily affect the B-wave. Familial foveal schisis has been reported in women [4].

Tapetoretinal Dystrophies

Leber's Congenital Amaurosis See previous discussion of this disorder.

Sector Retinitis Pigmentosa Retinitis pigmentosa is a genetically determined group of disorders associated with progressive degeneration of the retina which typically begins 360 degrees in the peripheral fundus. In some patients, only a sector of the retina is affected. Those patients with only the

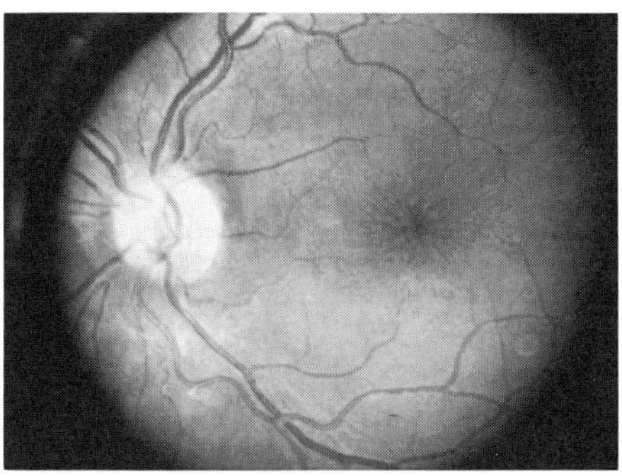

Figure 16 *Sex-linked juvenile retinoschisis showing typical foveomacular schisis.*

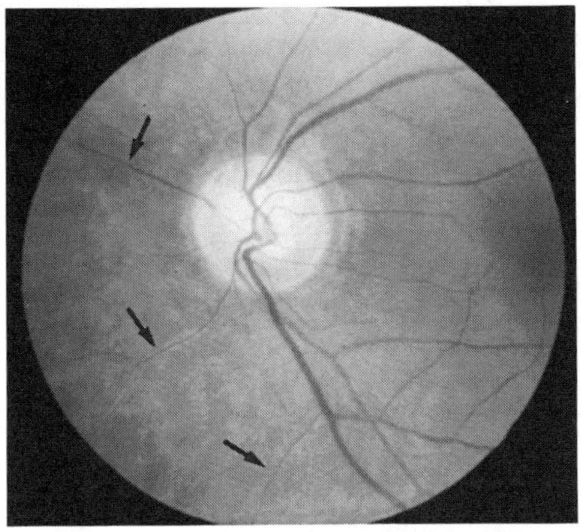

Figure 17 *Sector retinitis pigmentosa causing bitemporal visual field defect. Note pigment epithelial depigmentation and narrowing of retinal vessels* (arrows) *on the nasal side of the disc. The macula is normal. (From [4]. Used with permission.)*

nasal retina involved may complain of a bitemporal hemianopia and may be subjected to studies looking for chiasmatic lesions (Fig 17) [4]. Angiography may be helpful in delineating the affected segments by virtue of the hyperfluorescence associated with depigmentation of the pigment epithelium not evident by ophthalmoscopic examination.

Cerebral Macular Dystrophy—the "Neurolipidoses"

Neurolipidoses are neuronal storage diseases that can be divided into two broad types, the sphingolipidoses and the nonglycolipid neuronal storage disorders, or ceroid lipofuscinoses. In most cases, patients present early in life with clear-cut evidence of neurological disease associated with severe visual loss. Those with the sphingolipidoses often show evidence of a cherry-red spot in the macula. In some patients, particularly those with ceroid lipofuscinoses, onset of visual symptoms may not begin until childhood or early adulthood, and these symptoms may precede evidence of neurological involvement. Initially, the fundi of these patients may appear normal, but later, pigment epithelial degenerative changes occur that often begin in the macula and rapidly extend throughout the fundi.

Inflammatory Retinal Diseases

Multiple Evanescent White Dot Syndrome, Acute Idiopathic Blind Spot Enlargement Syndrome See previous discussion of these disorders.

Diffuse Unilateral Subacute Neuroretinitis See previous discussion of this disorder.

Toxic Retinopathy

There are multiple causes of toxic degeneration of the retina and optic nerve. Although the history of exposure to the toxic agent is often available, patients may fail either intentionally or unintentionally to give such a history. In many instances the fundi may appear normal during the early stages of visual loss.

Chloroquine Retinopathy Some patients who have received chloroquine for a total dose of between 100 and 300 gm may develop loss of central or paracentral vision that initially may be associated with minimal or no alterations in the pigment epithelium. Eventually, a bull's-eye pattern of depigmentation develops in the macular region.

Nicotinic Acid Maculopathy Patients taking 1.5 to 5 gm of nicotinic acid per day may develop bilateral loss of central vision that is associated with a peculiar nonfluorescein-staining cystoid macular edema [18]. They experience rapid recovery of vision after discontinuing the nicotinic acid.

Quinine Toxicity Quinine toxicity usually occurs with doses more than 4 gm but may occur with smaller doses. Patients may develop nausea, vomiting, and tinnitis and may become obtunded or comatose. On awakening, they may be totally blind with a normal appearing fundus. The fluorescein angiogram shows minimal loss of background choroidal fluorescein, and an electrooculogram usually shows no light rise [19]. Within several days patients often recover normal central acuity but retain only a small island of central vision. Progressive narrowing of the retinal arteries and pallor of the optic disc begins within several days.

Methyl Alcohol Toxicity These patients experience symptoms varying from spots in front of the eyes to complete blindness usually within 18 to 48 hours after ingestion of methyl alcohol. They show varying degrees of pupillary light reflex impairment, which is of considerable prognostic significance. Those with dilated fixed pupils usually die or experience severe permanent visual damage. Ophthalmoscopic examination may show hyperemia and edema of the optic disc with engorgement of the retinal veins. Those with severe damage will develop optic atrophy. A dense centrocecal scotoma sparing central fixation is the most frequent field defect.

Cancer-associated Retinopathy Patients with carcinoma that is often occult may develop rapid loss of vision associated with nyctalopia, ring scotoma, and a flat electroretinographic response, which initially may be associated with minimal or no ophthalmoscopic changes [20]. Within several months they usually develop signs of some arterial narrowing.

Nutritional Amblyopia Patients may experience progressive loss of central vision associated with a centrocecal visual field defect caused by dietary deficiency of one or several vitamins. Visual loss is initially unassociated with fundus change, but optic disc pallor, particularly temporally, usually develops. Most patients, during the early stages of visual loss, will show improvement of vision following restitution of a balanced diet and B-complex vitamin supplementation.

Senile Retinoschisis and Rhegmatogenous Detachment

Segmental visual field defects may be caused by unrecognized rhegmatogenous retinal detachment (relative field defect) or retinoschisis (absolute field defect). Their ophthalmoscopic detection may be particularly difficult in patients who have either a shallow retinal detachment or schisis, or in whom spontaneous retinal reattachment or collapse of the schisis has occurred. Fluorescein angiography is helpful in identifying the area of chronic shallow retinal detachment that will be evident as a zone of hyperfluorescence caused by the depigmentation of the pigment epithelium.

■ References

1. Byrne SF, Glaser JS. Orbital tissue differentiation with standardized echography. Ophthalmology 1983;90:1071–1090
2. Hupp SL, Buckley EG, Byrne SF, et al. Posttraumatic venous stasis obstructive retinopathy associated with enlarged optic nerve sheath. Arch Ophthalmol 1984; 102:254–256
3. Sergott RC, Cohen MS, Bosley TM, et al. Optic nerve decompression may improve the progressive form of nonarteritic ischemic optic neuropathy. Arch Ophthalmol 1989;107:1743–1754
4. Gass JDM. Stereoscopic atlas of macular diseases. Diagnosis and treatment. St. Louis: CV Mosby, 1987, pp 235–765
5. Gass JDM, Braunstein RA. Sessile and exophytic capillary angiomas of the juxtapapillary retina and optic nerve head. Arch Ophthalmol 1980;98:1790–1797
6. Cotlier E. Cafe-au-lait spots of the fundus in neurofibromatosis. Arch Ophthalmol 1977;95:1990–1992
7. Wallace DC, Singh G, Lott MT, et al. Mitochondrial DNA mutation associated with Leber's hereditary optic neuropathy. Science 1988;242:1427–1430
8. Flynn JT, Cullen RF. Disc oedema in congenital amaurosis of Leber. Br J Ophthalmol 1975;59:497–502
9. Dreyer RF, Hopen G, Gass JDM, Smith JL. Leber's idiopathic stellate neuroretinitis. Arch Ophthalmol 1984;102:1140–1145
10. Gass JDM, Braunstein RA. Further observations concerning the diffuse unilateral subacute neuroretinitis syndrome. Arch Ophthalmol 1983;101:1689–1697
11. Brinton GS, Osher RH, Gass JDM. Idiopathic vitritis. Retina 1983;3:95–98
12. Gass JDM. Vitiliginous chorioretinitis. Arch Ophthalmol 1981;99:1778–1787
13. Dreyer RF, Gass JDM. Multifocal choroiditis and panuveitis; a syndrome that mimics ocular histoplasmosis. Arch Ophthalmol 1984;102:1776–1784
14. Jampol LM, Sieving PA, Pugh D, et al. Multiple evanescent white dot syndrome. I. Clinical findings. Arch Ophthalmol 1984;102:671–674
15. Fletcher WA, Imes RK, Goodman D, et al. Acute idiopathic blind spot enlargement: a big blind spot syndrome without optic disc edema. Arch Ophthalmol 1988; 106:440–449
16. Barr CC, Glaser JS, Blankenship G. Acute disc swelling in juvenile diabetes. Clinical profile and natural history in 12 cases. Arch Ophthalmol 1980;98:2185–2192
17. Miller NR. Walsh and Hoyt's clinical neuro-ophthalmology, 4th ed. Baltimore: Williams & Wilkins, 1982:222–223
18. Gass JDM. Nicotinic acid maculopathy. Am J Ophthalmol 1973;76:500–510
19. Brinton GS, Norton EWD, Zahn JR, Knighton RW. Ocular quinine toxicity. Am J Ophthalmol 1980;90:403–410
20. Keltner JL, Roth AM, Chang RS. Photoreceptor degeneration: possible autoimmune disorder. Arch Ophthalmol 1983;101:564–569

Magnetic Resonance Imaging Applications in Ophthalmology

John A. McCrary III, M.D.

The advent of computerized tomography (CT) in 1975 began a new era in imaging technology. The broad clinical applications of CT became immediately obvious. CT provided a new, more sensitive way to image soft tissue and bone. Prior to CT, the use of plain skull radiography, polytomography, arteriography, pneumoencephalography, and positive contrast ventriculography were, as a group, either diagnostically less sensitive than CT or had significant morbidity associated with their use. CT was quickly appreciated as safer and more convenient for specific diagnosis of many central nervous system disorders.

Yet another breakthrough in imaging technology was realized with the introduction of magnetic resonance imaging (MRI). During the early 1980s it became apparent that this imaging technique might have the capability to surpass the advances of CT. Patient safety was identified as an immediate benefit, because MRI does not use ionizing radiation to produce images of body tissue. MRI is now accepted as the most sensitive, and among the most specific, diagnostic imaging tools available for most neuro-ophthalmic applications.

The purpose of this chapter is to acquaint practicing clinicians with the advantages and pitfalls of MRI for the diagnosis of some conditions that may be encountered in clinical practice. The applications of MRI are discussed by anatomical regions of disease rather than a complete list of diseases that might be found in any specific location. The advantages and disadvantages of MRI are compared with those of CT where appropriate. Current advances in MRI methods will be emphasized. Three recently published papers detail many of the conditions described [1–3].

MRI Production

Principles

Detailed descriptions of the physical characteristics of MRI are reported elsewhere. Only the basics will be considered here.

Hydrogen atoms, widely distributed in body water, spin in a random fashion. The spin of the single electron around the proton core of a hydrogen atom generates a small magnetic field. Because spin is random, the net magnetic field of all mobile hydrogen atoms in the body is zero.

If body tissue is introduced into an environment with a strong magnetic field, hydrogen atoms align themselves in a unidirectional way. The net result is more or less uniform gyromagnetic direction. Subsequent introduction of a radio-frequency pulse across a tissue bed that has had protons aligned via an external magnetic field can cause the net proton spin to be moved from the prestimulus direction of alignment to a new one. The net change in spin direction during and after radio-frequency stimulation generates a net electromagnetic signal change. This signal difference can be recorded, analyzed by computer, and an image can be made from this data. These are the principles involved in MRI.

Certain specific radio frequencies and pulse sequences can be used to best define the neuroanatomy of the soft tissue parts within the image field. Other radio-frequency pulse trains can be used to enhance the contrast between diseased and normal tissue within that field. T1-weighted images are used when a detailed study of the neuroanatomy of a particular region is desirable; T2-weighted images are more advantageous in defining regions of altered function caused by disease processes. To produce a T1-weighted image the radio-frequency pulse used has a short TE (echo time), and a short TR (relaxation time); often the TE is in the range of 25 msec, whereas the TR is 80 msec. T2-weighted images, on the contrary, require use of a long TE (80–100 msec) and a long TR (2 seconds or more). For quick reference, look at the eyes and ventricles on the MRIs. The ocular vitreous is dark as is the cerebrospinal fluid (CSF) contained in the cerebral ventricles on T1-weighted scan sections. Orbital fat is bright white. T2-weighted scans show bright, white CSF and vitreous with dark orbital fat. Exact sequence timing may vary in different imaging facilities depending on the type of equipment being used and the personal choice of the radiologist.

Spin (proton) density images can also be obtained as part of the study. These require use of a short TE and a long TR. Spin density images are generally of no greater value than good T1- and T2-weighted images for most applications.

Disturbances in blood-brain barrier function are often recognizable as areas of disease in T2-weighted images. Techniques are now available to emphasize regions of blood-brain barrier disturbance in T1-weighted scans by using paramagnetic substances such as gadolinium, which will be described.

MRI scans image mobile protons far better than those protons that are fixed in a rigid system with low water content, which is the reason MRI is not usually helpful to study disease states of cranial bone. CT is far more useful.

Enhancement Techniques

Enhancement techniques can be used to alter T1 relaxation. Use of paramagnetic substances such as iron, manganese, and gadolinium have been used for this purpose. The only clinically valuable enhancement agent currently approved for human use is gadolinium DPTA [4]. This agent is safe; it is normally administered intravenously. It can be used to identify regions within the orbit or central nervous system with defective blood-brain barrier function

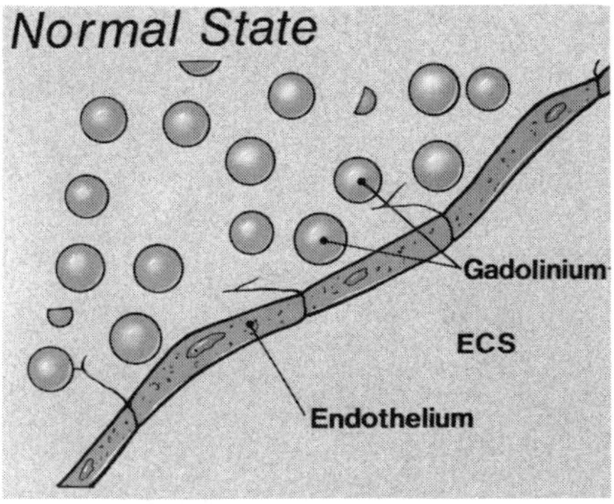

Figure 1 *Normal physiological state after gadolinium contrast is injected intravenously. The contrast agent does not leak through the vascular endothelium into the surrounding tissue* (ECS).

(Figs 1, 2). As contrast leaks through the defective blood-brain barrier into the surrounding tissue, the T1 soft tissue image will appear bright, rather than the normal gray color.

Image Planes and Strategies

MRI can be obtained in any desired plane without the need to reposition the patient as is required for high-quality CT scanning. Any scan plane can be generated from instructions typed at the computer keyboard (Fig 3). The fact that patients do not need to be moved is an advantage over CT. A strategic approach to MRI based on each clinical problem is more cost-effective and diagnostically accurate [5]. A clinically driven imaging scheme is more productive because the impaired neuroanatomical region receives special attention.

Patient Acceptance

Putting a patient into an MRI scanner may cause significant claustrophobia. In fact, this is one disadvantage of MRI. Nearly 30% of the individuals brought to the MRI facility will complain of feeling "closed in, in a coffin, or about to go crazy" because of the body confinement within the long bore of the magnet. Additionally, patients complain of noise while the test is in progress. These problems may necessitate patient sedation to complete an MRI study. If these issues are not identified and controlled before imaging is well

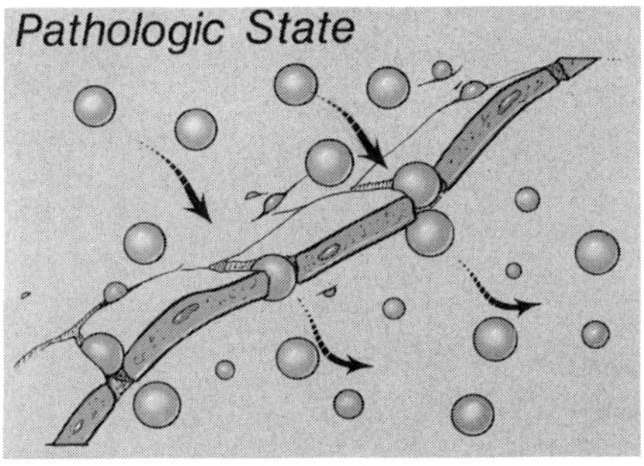

Figure 2 *When a pathological condition occurs, the vascular endothelium is often damaged. This damage can permit gadolinium to leak into the extravascular compartment.*

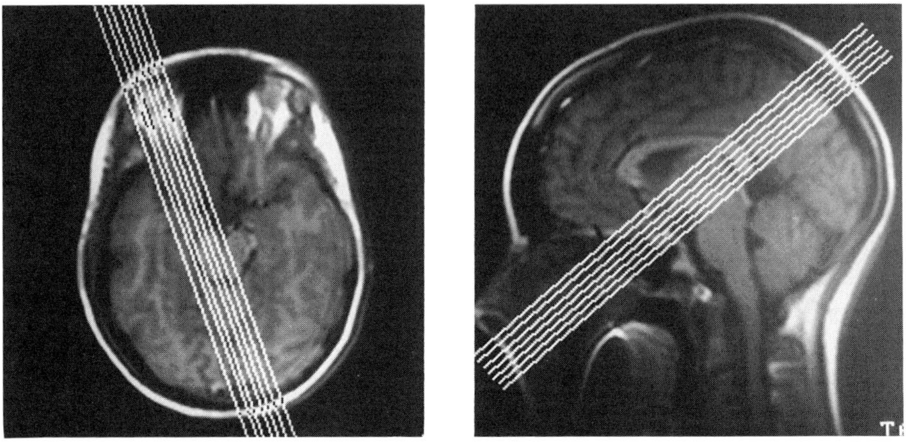

A B

Figure 3 *(A) Parasagittal orientation lines used to delineate the axes of magnetic resonance imaging slices used to evaluate a right-sided optic nerve tumor. (B) Orientation of axial scan sections to be taken for an optic nerve tumor. Sections are optimized to reveal any evidence of intracranial tumor extension.*

along, motion artifact is sure to produce a very poor result caused by an anxious, moving patient.

■ MRI of Eye, Optic Nerve, and Orbit

Debate continues regarding the advantages and disadvantages of MRI as opposed to CT when looking at diseases of the eye, optic nerve, and orbit. There are a number of reasons for this debate. In trauma patients, particularly where a foreign body or a fracture might be a significant consideration, MRI would be disadvantageous because the strong magnetic field could produce movement of an unsuspected magnetic foreign body. Furthermore, MRI does not image bone well. Therefore, fractures are invisible unless there is bony displacement. For these reasons, one should initially rely on CT in most patients with orbital trauma.

Ocular tumor can be imaged by both techniques. Both CT and MRI can identify large intraocular tumors such as choroidal melanoma or retinoblastoma [6–7]. CT may be superior to MRI with respect to retinoblastoma because the CT can better image calcium deposits within the tumor. MRI may or may not show flecks of calcium as tiny, black voids within the tumor bed. MRI may be better than CT for the diagnosis of choroidal melanoma, because the melanin can cause a paramagnetic effect that may cause a bright signal to appear within the tumor. Melanin, or the iron contained in hemoglobin, causes excessive T1 relaxation as compared with normal surrounding soft tissue. Tissue containing either will have an abnormally bright signal. MRI can also successfully image ocular lesions other than tumors [8]. These lesions include intra-

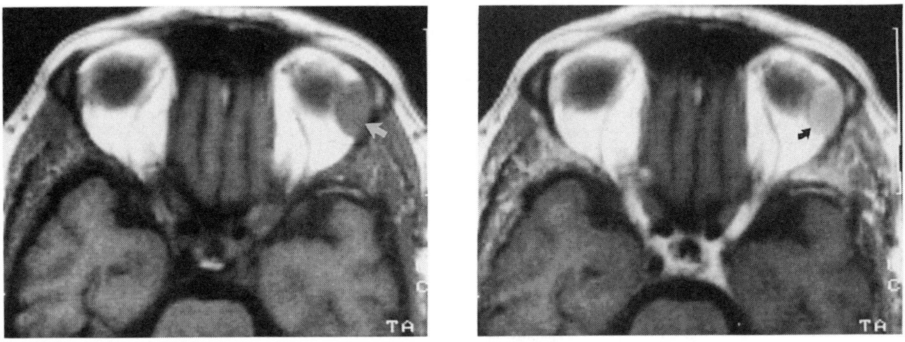

A B

Figure 4 *(A) Axial, T1-weighted, unenhanced orbital magnetic resonance imaging section demonstrates a left lacrimal gland tumor* (arrow). *(B) After gadolinium enhancement. The medial wall of the gland does not enhance* (arrow) *and can be differentiated from the tumor.*

ocular blood, vitreous opacities, retinal detachment, and various ocular deformities.

Inflammatory diseases of the orbit, including pseudotumor [9], orbital myositis, and thyroid ophthalmopathy [10] can be imaged satisfactorily with MRI, but motion artifact may cause substandard images to be obtained. If patients cannot remain still long enough to ensure good quality, CT is a better choice. In most orbital inflammatory conditions I usually choose CT over MRI because image quality is usually excellent, cost is reduced, acquisition time is short, and bony detail can be readily appreciated.

Orbital and optic nerve tumors can be well identified with both CT and MRI. For most orbital tumors, CT is quite adequate, particularly with respect to lacrimal gland tumors (Fig 4) when the differentiation of benign mixed tumor from lacrimal gland carcinoma hinges in large part on the bony anatomy of the lacrimal fossa. Orbital tumors such as capillary hemangioma, neurofibroma, and lymphoma can usually be equally well defined with CT as with MRI [11].

Tumors of the optic nerve present specific imaging challenges. The two most common tumors encountered in the optic nerve are optic nerve glioma [12] (Fig 5) and meningioma [13] of the optic nerve sheath (Fig 6). Both of these tumors require detailed assessment of the intracranial and intracanalicular portion of the optic nerve. The best management of patients who have unilateral disease and no apparent clinical indication of extension of tumor into the optic chiasm may depend on the quality of images taken of the prechiasmatic segment of the optic nerves. Usually MRI provides the best assessment of the intracranial portion of the optic nerve. In most patients with optic nerve tumor, MRI is the preferred first study. There are occasions when contrast-enhanced CT scans of the optic nerve may be better, compared to MRIs, when presurgical planning is under way. For the majority of patients, however, MRI is the superior study. The use of gadolinium enhancement is valuable to facilitate MRI diagnosis of optic nerve sheath meningioma. Small meningiomas

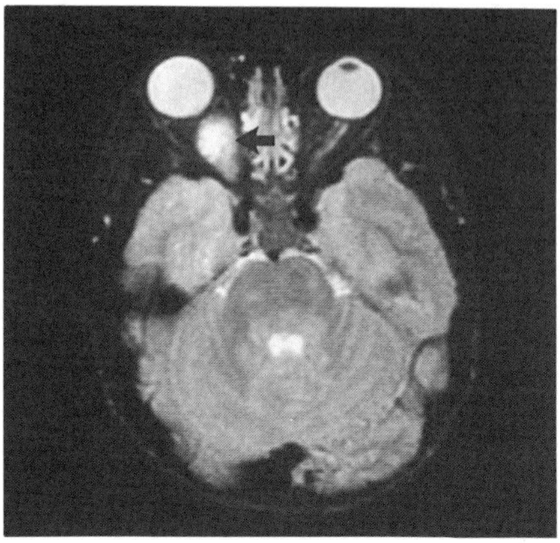

Figure 5 *T2-weighted, unenhanced, axial magnetic resonance imaging section demonstrates the typical fusiform enlargement of an optic nerve glioma* (arrow). *The fellow optic nerve is normal.*

within the sheath can be invisible if gadolinium is not used. CT may fail to demonstrate these tumors if iodinated contrast is not used.

Inflammatory or infiltrative diseases of the optic nerve such as sarcoid or metastatic neoplasm are often better imaged with MRI than with CT [14, 15]. Disease at the orbital apex may require comparison CT to obtain sophisticated views of bony anatomy that may help distinguish the extent or type of disease. Therefore, patients with optic nerve tumors such as meningioma or glioma and those with possible sarcoidosis or other infiltrative diseases often require complementary CT to visualize bony detail before making a final decision about management.

Except for the applications discussed, MRI is probably no better than CT

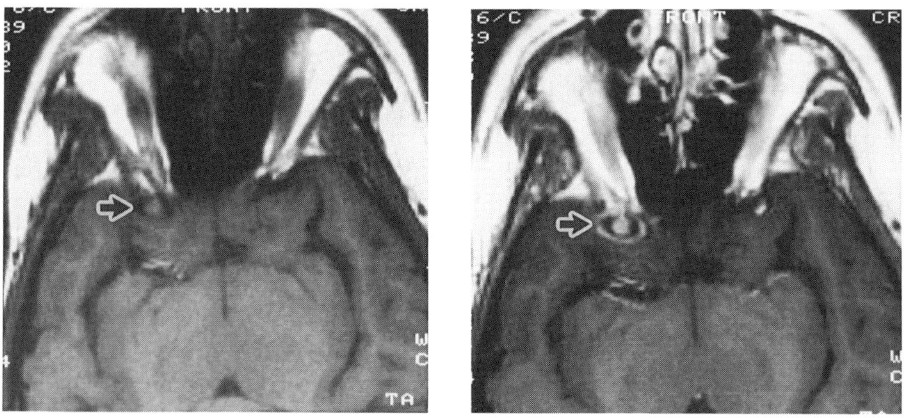

A B

Figure 6 *(A) T1-weighted, axial, unenhanced magnetic resonance imaging section through the intracranial segment of an optic nerve meningioma* (arrow) *reveals little evidence of disease. (B) After injection of intravenous gadolinium, there is evidence of intracranial tumor extension* (arrow).

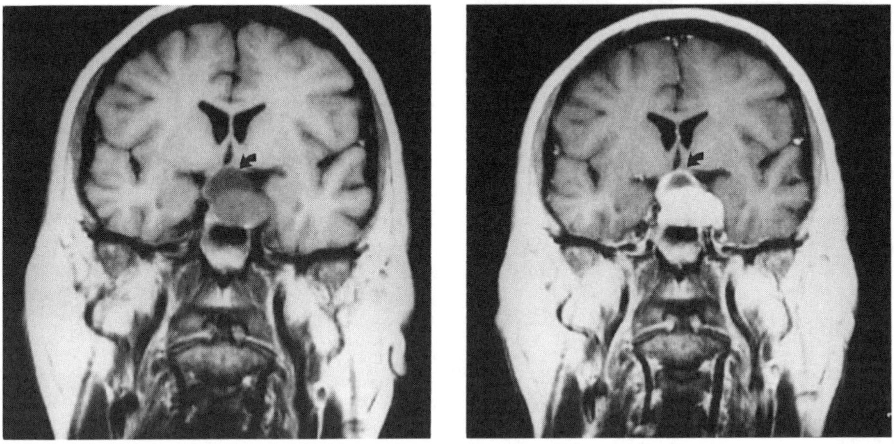

A B

Figure 7 *(A) Coronal, T1-weighted, enhanced magnetic resonance imaging section through a pituitary tumor showing both solid and cystic components. The cystic component with its boundary zone of capsule is in contact with the optic chiasm* (arrow). *(B) Following gadolinium enhancement, the rostral extent of the tumor capsule and its relationship to the optic chiasm* (arrow) *is more clearly imaged.*

for imaging of ocular or orbital disease in the majority of patients. Compromised image quality caused by motion artifact remains a significant problem with MRI, especially as applied to diagnosis of orbital diseases.

■ Sella, Optic Chiasm, and Optic Tract Lesions

If disease is suspected in the intracranial compartment, MRI is the best imaging technique to use for virtually all soft tissue applications, especially when there is disease of the sella, suprasellar space, optic chiasm, or optic tract. MRI is the preferred first study unless the possibility of a metastatic or malignant primary neoplasm is being considered. Such tumors are uncommon. Pituitary tumors [16], optic chiasmal gliomas [17], craniopharyngiomas, and meningiomas that are commonly encountered are readily identifiable with quality axial and coronal thin-section MRI [18], particularly when gadolinium is introduced to define boundaries between normal and affected tissue (Figs 7, 8). Meningiomas within the parasellar region may be totally missed if gadolinium is not used. Contrast-enhanced MRI scans should be routinely obtained when this area is being studied.

The mark of a high-quality MRI scan of the optic chiasmal region is visualization of the pituitary stalk, unless it is surrounded by abnormal tissue. At least one coronal section MRI slice should reveal the pituitary stalk if the scan has been done properly. Parasagittal cuts taken off axis to the midline are also very helpful in determining the lateral extent of tumor in the parasellar region and in the orbit. Sagittal and parasagittal sections are routinely obtained in the individuals we image with suspected parasellar lesions. Identification of bony

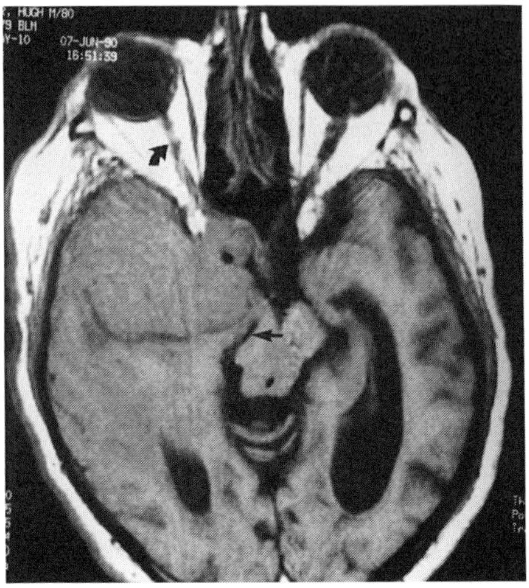

Figure 8 *Unenhanced axial, T1-weighted MR section showing the anatomy of the optic nerves. Atrophy of the right optic nerve* (curved arrow) *caused by chronic compression from a large meningioma is seen. There is also effacement and lateral displacement of the right ventral surface of the midbrain at the level of the cerebral peduncle caused by posterior-lateral pressure from the tumor* (straight arrow).

recontouring or demineralization caused by a suspected metastatic process or intrinsic calcification within the tumor of a craniopharyngioma will be better demonstrated by CT. With the exception of these clinical situations, MRI is the preferred initial imaging study.

It is important to remember that the optic tracts will not be well visualized unless special scan planes are obtained to identify these structures. If disease in or around the optic tract is suspected, the imaging team should be made aware of this suspicion to idealize the scan sections to maximally reveal the anatomy. Infarctions, tumor compression, or demyelination of the optic tract can be readily identified if appropriate attention to detail is observed. The same applies to a lesion of the lateral geniculate body that can be a very rare cause of homonymous hemianopia.

Cerebral Hemispheres

Postgeniculate visual radiations can be best studied with MRI. You should try to be as specific as possible in guiding the neuroradiologist to the probable location of disease based on your assessment of the patient's visual acuity, pupils, visual fields, and ophthalmoscopic examination. Any of the diseases mentioned can, and often do, affect other areas of the brain. These diseases are discussed here because the cerebral hemispheres are so often involved.

MRI is far superior to CT for early identification of cerebrovascular accidents [19], the changes associated with multiple sclerosis [20, 21], vasculitis, metastatic neoplasm, primary neoplasm [22], and a host of other conditions (Fig 9). From a practical standpoint, if a patient with an unexplained hemianopic visual field defect is being investigated, MRI is the preferred technique. For example, one of the difficulties with CT scanning in early stroke is the problem of isodense infarction. CT is not nearly as sensitive in detecting early stroke as is MRI. MRI is the primary imaging procedure if patients are cooperative. With stroke, gadolinium enhancement is not routinely required. If neo-

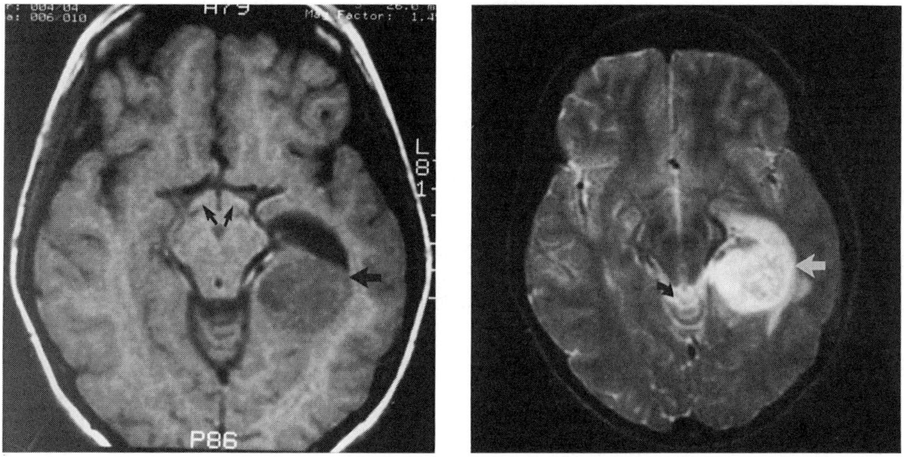

A B

Figure 9 *(A) T1-weighted, unenhanced axial magnetic resonance image of a large temporal lobe neoplasm* (large arrow) *reveals both solid and cystic components. The anterior half of the optic tracts are visible but not affected* (small arrow). *(B) T2-weighted study reveals boundary between the lesion* (large arrow) *and surrounding normal structures. Normal cerebrospinal fluid signal* (curved arrow) *over the cerebellar vermis and behind the dorsal midbrain should not be confused with the tumor.*

plastic disease is suspected, gadolinium enhancement is used to clearly define the tumor boundary from surrounding normal tissue. The use of gadolinium to try to differentiate active from inactive demyelination caused by multiple sclerosis has not yet been proved beneficial.

■ Posterior Fossa

Any study of brainstem structures, whether mesencephalic, pontine, or medullary will be better obtained by MRI. CT is of limited value in examining the posterior fossa due to beam-hardening artifact of the surrounding bone. For this reason, CT does not image small lesions in the posterior fossa as well as MRI. If clinical evaluation suggests the possibility of a posterior fossa lesion, patients should be imaged first with enhanced MRI.

Clinically, midbrain disease is characterized by bilateral slowing of pupillary reactions to light, limitation of vertical gaze on command, and defective convergence. These and other signs such as retraction convergence nystagmus and pathological retraction of the upper lids (Collier's sign) are features of dorsal midbrain syndrome. Clinical variations of midbrain disease include nuclear third nerve palsy and the Weber-Benedickt syndrome; the latter is characterized by ipsilateral third nerve palsy combined with contralateral hemiparesis or hemidyskinesia.

Because the fourth nerve also originates in the midbrain, fourth nerve palsy may be a sign of midbrain disease. Any patient with nystagmus, abnor-

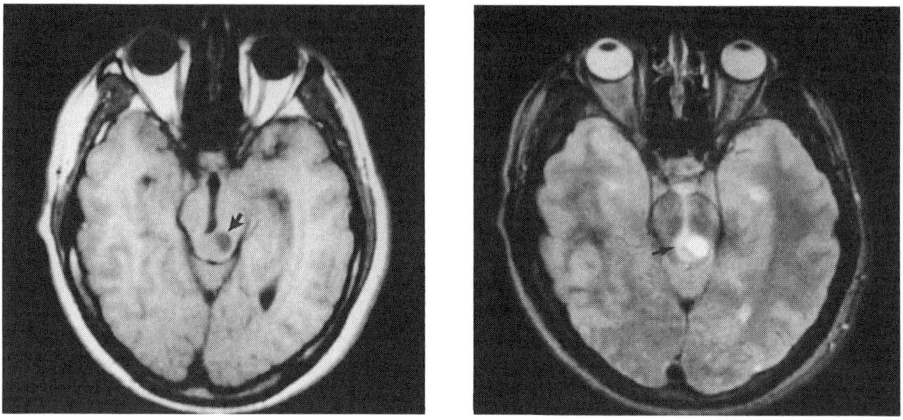

A B

Figure 10 *(A) Axial, T1-weighted, unenhanced magnetic resonance imaging section through the rostral brainstem showing a cystic neoplasm that occupies the dorsal midbrain* (arrow). *Soft tissue thickening and effacement of the left posterior aspect of the brainstem by this lesion is obvious. The patient had upgaze paresis, convergence-retraction nystagmus, and diminished pupillary constriction to light stimulation. (B) Axial T2-weighted scan better demonstrates the extension of the tumor across the midline* (arrow).

mally slow pupil reactions to light, and vertical gaze limitation should be imaged first with MRI [23, 24] (Fig 10). Dorsal midbrain syndrome is usually caused by neoplasm in young patients or ischemic disease in the elderly. Trauma and demyelinating disease can also cause dorsal midbrain syndrome.

Pontine disease often features dysfunction of cranial nerves five, six, seven, and eight, as well as nystagmus, conjugate gaze palsy, or paresis in the horizontal plane. Any combination of these signs suggests pontine brainstem disease. A detailed description of all the clinical permutations of pontine disease is not possible here, but, as an example, a patient who presents with a Bell's palsy (peripheral facial nerve palsy) combined with nystagmus, ipsilateral hearing loss, ataxia, and decreased facial sensation would be expected to have a lesion in the ipsilateral pons or adjacent cerebellopontine angle. Clinical suspicion of pontine dysfunction should cause clinicians to order MRI of the posterior fossa with special attention to the pons [25] (Fig 11). The pons and cerebellum will be much better imaged by MRI than by any other technique available. Preenhancement and postenhancement images should be routinely obtained in all patients, except those with a clear prescan etiology such as cerebrovascular ischemia. This practice actually saves money because repeat scans with gadolinium done later are time-consuming and add more cost than is the case when enhancement is done in the original study. Cerebrovascular accident, multiple sclerosis, inflammatory disease, and metastatic carcinoma can all be much better imaged by MRI than CT. Axial, coronal, and parasagittal cuts through damaged structures help identify extent of the disease.

Lesions of the medulla and foramen magnum can cause impairment of swallowing and gag reflex, dysphonia (hoarseness), weakness of shoulder eleva-

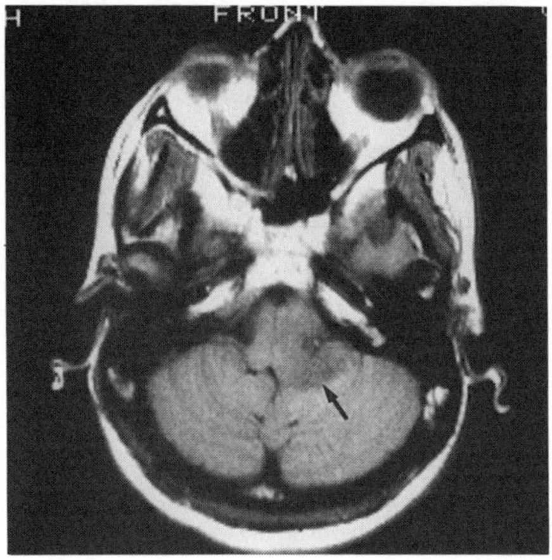

Figure 11 *An axial, T1-weighted magnetic resonance imaging section taken through the brainstem at the pontine level reveals a large neoplasm extending posterior and laterally into the cerebellum* (arrow). *This lesion did not show enhancement after contrast was injected. It is presumed to be a low-grade astrocytic tumor.*

tion, weakness of the tongue (protrusion), ataxia, and facial numbness. These findings can occur in many different combinations. One of the more common clinical presentations of medullary disease is the lateral medullary plate syndrome (Wallenberg's syndrome). This syndrome usually occurs in elderly patients who have a history of vascular disease. The clinical features include acute onset of ipsilateral facial numbness, Horner's syndrome, contralateral loss of pain and temperature sensation in the arm and leg, profound nystagmus, ataxia, nausea, vomiting, and skew deviation. Wallenberg's syndrome is caused by infarction within the area supplied by the posterior inferior cerebellar artery or one of its major branches.

Patients who come to ophthalmologists complaining of blurred vision noted when looking down should be examined carefully for evidence of downbeat nystagmus. This sign points to disease at the level of the foramen magnum. Patients with this condition should undergo an MRI scan to look for herniation of posterior fossa contents into the cervical spinal canal (Arnold-Chiari malformation [26]). This diagnosis is readily made with MRI. Sagittal and parasagittal MRI sections at the level of the foramen magnum reveal the abnormality. Herniation of the cerebellar tonsils through the foramen magnum into the cervical spinal canal is diagnostic. Gadolinium enhancement is not required unless one is suspicious of a tumor as the cause of downbeat nystagmus.

MRI is clearly the best imaging method to use for any of the posterior fossa disease processes described. Gadolinium enhancement is very helpful if a tumor is suspected, but it is not required for all of the conditions described. Supplementary cerebral arteriography may be indicated if patients have had a stroke.

■ Cavernous Sinus

The cavernous sinus lies just lateral to the pituitary fossa and is the convergence point for several neural structures that are important to ocular function.

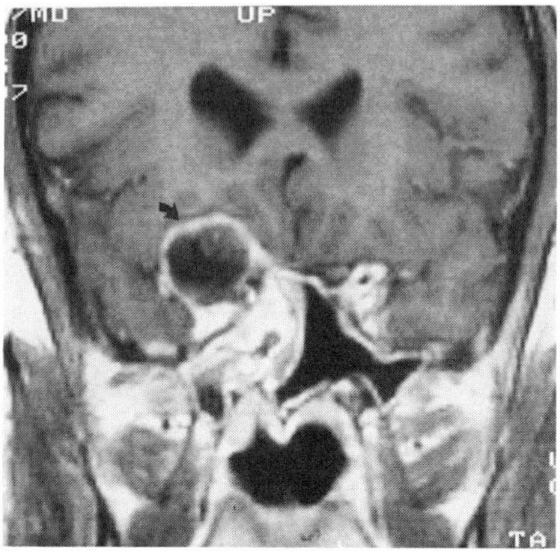

A

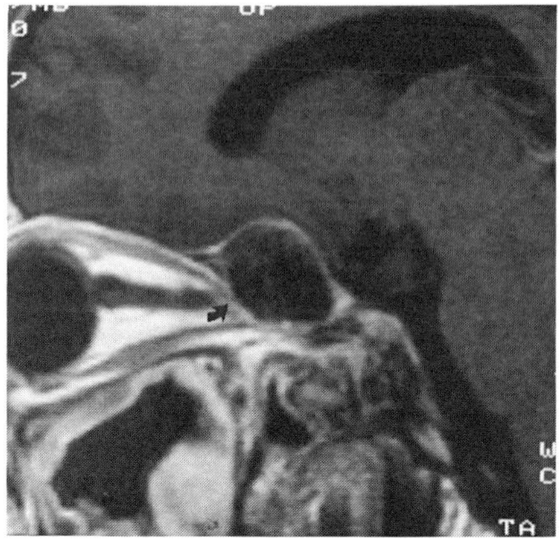

B

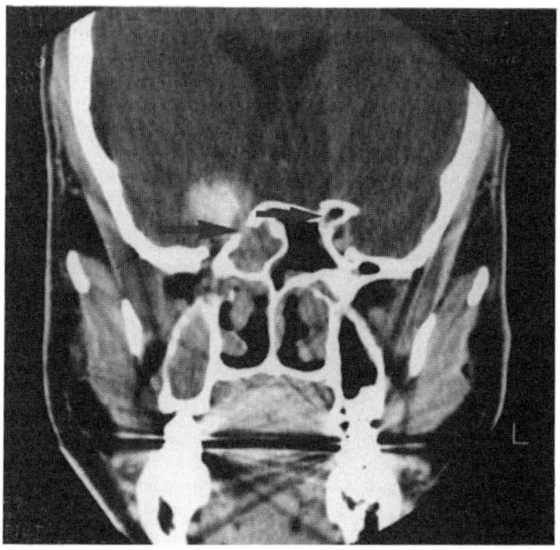

C

Figure 12 *(A) Coronal, T1-weighted, enhanced magnetic resonance imaging section through the parasellar region of a young man with headaches and a subacute, incomplete right-sided third nerve palsy revealing a large cystic lesion that occupies the cavernous sinus* (arrow). *The lesion is contiguous with the subadjacent, medial sphenoethmoidal sinus complex. The final diagnosis was mucocele; it was surgically removed. Full clinical recovery followed. (B) A parasagittal, off-axis, T1-weighted MR section showing the relationship of the mucocele to the orbital apex and optic nerve* (curved arrow). *(C) Coronal computed tomographic scan of the mucocele reveals destruction of the anterior clinoid process and the lateral wall of the sphenoid sinus* (large arrow). *For comparison, the normal left anterior clinoid can be seen* (small arrow).

The sixth cranial nerve courses through the sinus lateral to the carotid siphon as it passes forward toward the superior orbital fissure and orbit. Cranial nerves III and IV lie in the lateral wall of the sinus along with the first and second divisions of the trigeminal nerve. All of these nerves converge at the orbital apex. Around the carotid sheath, the sympathetic fibers pass forward toward the eye. A lesion of the cavernous sinus may produce weakness or paralysis of cranial nerves III, IV, V_1, V_2, VI, and in Horner's syndrome. These combinations vary. Occasionally, an isolated palsy of one of these cranial nerves will be caused by a lesion of the intracavernous or paracavernous region (Fig 12).

If there is suspicion of a possible cavernous sinus lesion, MRI is usually a better choice than CT unless bony detail along the floor of the skull must be seen. For example, if you suspect nasopharyngeal carcinoma or metastatic tumor invasion of the cavernous sinus, CT may be helpful because destruction of bone in the skull base is commonly seen with these conditions.

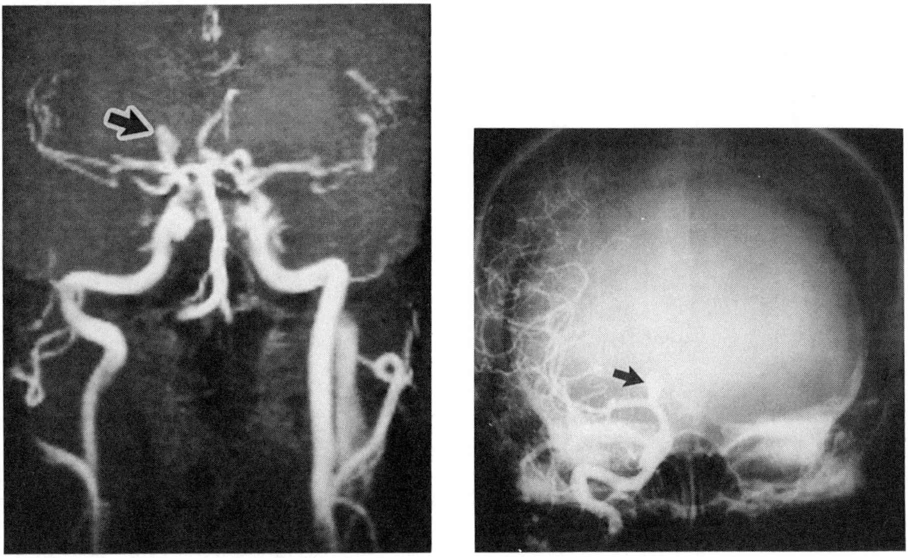

A B

Figure 13 *(A) Magnetic resonance (MR) angiogram shows a right middle cerebral artery aneurysm* (arrow). *(B) Standard cerebral arteriogram reveals little additional detail about the size or shape of the aneurysm* (arrow) *when compared to the MR study. (Courtesy of Marlin E. Sandlin, M.D.)*

The most common lesions found in the cavernous sinus are meningioma and intracavernous carotid aneurysm, although inflammatory conditions such as Tolosa-Hunt syndrome may occur [27]. High-quality axial and coronal MRIs are needed first. Gadolinium enhancement is useful for all soft tissue tumors of the cavernous sinus. Supplemented by CT scans, cerebral arteriography, and spinal fluid investigation, most diseases that affect the cavernous sinus and superior orbital fissure can be diagnosed accurately.

■ MRI Developing Techniques

Among the most exciting of the evolving technologies are MRI cerebral angiography and surface coil recording of orbital or ocular lesions. MRI angiography uses specialized software that permits data manipulation so as to blur the parenchymal soft tissue images of the brain and orbits yet idealize the images obtained from the blood columns within cerebral and extracranial arteries. The capability now exists to clearly identify the major branches of the extracranial and intracranial carotid and vertebrobasilar systems. Aneurysms of 3.0 mm [28] or more can be readily appreciated on MRI angiography as can major obstruction of blood flow. This totally noninvasive imaging method is especially suited to investigation of high-risk patients prior to consideration of cerebral angiography (Fig 13). The technique does not require contrast enhancement.

Surface coil design and use continues to improve the detail that can be achieved on MRI assessment of the eye and orbit. Furthermore, spectroscopic methods using surface coil recording show promise for evaluation of altered metabolic activity within regions of damaged brain tissue.

■ References

1. Kwan ES. Radiologic evaluation of neuro-ophthalmologic disease. Curr Opin Ophthalmol 1990;1:484–498
2. Jay WM. Advances in magnetic resonance imaging. Am J Ophthalmol 1989;108: 592–596
3. Slamovits TL, Gardner TA. Neuroimaging in neuro-ophthalmology. Ophthalmology 1989;96:555–568
4. Bronen RA, Sze G. Magnetic resonance imaging contrast agents: theory and application to the nervous system. J Neurosurg 1990;73:820–839
5. Hyman RA, Gorey MT. Imaging strategies for MR of the brain. Radiol Clin North Am 1988;26:471–503
6. Peyster RG, Augsburger JJ, Shields JA, et al. Intraocular tumors: evaluation with MR imaging. Radiology 1988;168:773–779
7. Mafee MF, Goldberg MF, Greenwald MJ, et al. Retinoblastoma and simulating lesions: role of CT and MR imaging. Radiol Clin North Am 1987;25:667–682
8. Tonami H, Tamamura H, Kimizu K, et al. Intraocular lesions in patients with systemic disease: findings on MR imaging. AJNR 1989;10:1185–1189
9. Atlas SW, Grossman RI, Savino PJ, et al. Surface-coil MR of orbital pseudotumor. AJR Am J Roentgenol 1987;148:803–808
10. Hosten N, Sander B, Cordes M, et al. Graves' ophthalmopathy: MR imaging of the orbits. Radiology 1989;172:759–762
11. Mafee MF, Putterman A, Valvassori GE, et al. Orbital space-occupying lesions: role of computed tomography and magnetic resonance imaging. Radiol Clin North Am 1987;25:529–559
12. Haik BG, Saint-Louis L, Bierly J, et al. Magnetic resonance imaging in the evaluation of optic nerve gliomas. Ophthalmology 1987;94:709–717
13. Hendrix LE, Kneeland JB, Haughton VM, et al. MR imaging of optic nerve lesions: value of gadopentetate dimeglumine and fat-suppression techniques. Am J Roentgenol 1990;155:849–854
14. Daniels DL, Yu S, Pech P, et al. Computed tomography and magnetic resonance imaging of the orbital apex. Radiol Clin North Am 1987;25:803–817
15. Bilaniuk LT, Atlas SW, Zimmerman RA. Magnetic resonance imaging of the orbit. Radiol Clin North Am 1987;25:509–528
16. Davis PC, Hoffman JC, Spencer T, et al. MR imaging of the pituitary adenoma: CT, clinical and surgical correlation. AJR Am J Roentgenol 1987;148:797–802
17. Albert A, Lee BCP, Saint-Louis L, et al. MRI of optic chiasm and optic pathways. AJNR 1986;7:255–258
18. Naheedy MH, Haag JR, Azar-Kia B, et al. MRI and CT of sellar and parasellar disorders. Radiol Clin North Am 1987;25:819–847
19. Kinkel PR, Kinkel WR, Jacobs L. Nuclear magnetic resonance imaging in patients with stroke. Semin Neurol 1986;6:43–52
20. Uhlenbrock D, Sehlen S. The value of T-1 weighted images in the differentiation between MS, white matter lesions and subcortical arteriosclerotic encephalopathy (SAE). Neuroradiology 1989;31:203–212
21. Miller DH, Ormerod IEC, Gibson A, et al. MR scanning in patients with vasculitis: differentiation from multiple sclerosis. Neuroradiology 1987;29:226–231

22. Higer HP, Pedrosa P, Schuth M. MR imaging of cerebral tumors: state of the art and work in progress. Neurosurg Rev 1989;12:91–106
23. Tien RD, Barkovich AJ, Edwards MSB. MR imaging of pineal tumors. AJNR 1990;11:557–565
24. Barkhof F, Valk J. "Top of the basilar" syndrome: comparison of clinical and MR findings. Neuroradiology 1988;30:293–298
25. Ruff RL, Wiener SN, Leigh RJ. Magnetic resonance imaging in patients with diplopia. A review. Invest Radiol 1986;21:311–319
26. Bosley TM, Cohen DA, Schatz NJ, et al. Comparison of metrizamide computed tomography and magnetic resonance imaging in the evaluation of lesions at the cervicomedullary junction. Neurology 1985;35:485–492
27. Yousem DM, Atlas SW, Grossman RI, et al. MR imaging of Tolosa-Hunt syndrome. AJNR 1989;10:1181–1184
28. Ross JS, Masaryk TJ, Modic MT, et al. Intracranial aneurysms: evaluation by MR angiography. AJNR 1990;11:449–455

Botulinum Toxin Injections for Treatment of Blepharospasm and Hemifacial Spasm

Jonathan D. Wirtschafter, M.D., F.A.C.S.
Marian Rubenfeld, M.D., Ph.D.

History

Alan B. Scott, M.D., of San Francisco has investigated the use of botulinum toxin type A over the past 10 years (Oculinum; Oculinum Inc, San Francisco, CA) to weaken extraocular muscles and the orbicularis oculi muscles as an alternative to denervation or surgical weakening procedures [1]. "Botox" will be used generically throughout this chapter because the drug may be prepared differently in other countries. Prior to this approach, injections of alcohol and local anesthetics had been tried for similar purposes with unsatisfactory results. In December 1989 the Food and Drug Administration (FDA) approved use of the drug for eyelid spasms and strabismus in persons over the age of 12. Although Scott's original intention was to treat strabismus, Botox has found most acceptance in the treatment of muscle spasms. Although Botox is useful for certain extraocular muscle problems, so many other uses for Botox were under investigation that in November 1990 the National Institutes of Health convened a Consensus Development Conference on the Clinical Use of Botulinum Toxin [2]. Assessments of the clinical indications and uses have been prepared by the American Academies of Neurology and Ophthalmology [3, 4]. Some of the proposed nonophthalmic uses of Botox are listed in Table 1. We review the current status of Botox and other treatments used for treatment of eyelid spasms.

Description

Oculinum is a freeze-dried residue of botulinum toxin type A. The crystalline neurotoxin-hemagglutinin complex has a molecular weight of approximately 900 kd and is more stable than the neurotoxin alone, which is a single-chain protein with a molecular weight of approximately 150 kd. The neurotoxin is comprised of two chains designated as heavy and light, which, when dissociated, are nontoxic [5, 6]. The heavy chain binds to the receptors near the neuromuscular junctions of the lower motor neurons. The active site for tissue binding of the molecule may be a sialoglycoprotein. The biological

Table 1 *Nonophthalmological Uses of Botulinum Toxin*[a]

1. Idiopathic dystonias (adult-onset are usually focal or segmental; juvenile-onset are usually generalized)
2. Symptomatic dystonias associated with recognized hereditary neurological syndromes and quadriceps muscle spasms of multiple sclerosis
3. Dystonia due to environmental causes including drugs, toxins, and injuries
4. Detrusor sphincter dyssynergia following spinal cord injuries, anismus (idiopathic anal sphincter spasms)
5. Speech disorders including spastic dysphonia, stuttering, and laryngospasm [24]

[a]From [2].

action of the toxin advances with three sequential steps: membrane binding of the heavy chain, internalization of the light chain, and poisoning of intracellular processes. The light chain is attached at right angles near the middle of the heavy chain and enters the cell membrane, where it may act as an enzyme that inhibits the role of calcium ions in the release of acetylcholine. The toxin is inactivated by reducing the disulfide covalent that links the two chains. Botulinum toxin type A is serologically distinct from the other six toxins produced by *Clostridium botulinum* and related bacterial species. The toxins do not appear to have any internal role in the metabolism of the bacteria that synthesize them. Moreover, humans are not uniformly sensitive to each serotype of neurotoxin and are absolutely resistant to some of them.

The toxin is produced using seed stocks of Hall strain *C. botulinum* and sterile complex medium and fermented for approximately 72 hours, at which time bacterial lysis occurs. The protein is purified and stabilized by the addition of human serum albumin (0.5 mg/100 U) sterilized to prevent infection with hepatitis and human immunodeficiency viruses (HIV). The product is standardized and the toxicity and dosage are expressed as LD_{50} units for mice (LD_{50} is the lethal dose for 50% of mice of a certain weight).

■ Actions

Botox interferes with release of acetylcholine from nerve terminals and is thus a presynaptic blocking agent for cholinergic junctions and a neuromuscular blocker for efferent fibers to skeletal muscles. It is known that Botox acts on individual terminals because not all fibers in one motor unit fail at one time. Botox might have the ability to act on individual neurons in the central nervous system, but it cannot penetrate the blood-brain barrier. Botox causes no electrophysiological effects on the electroretinogram of rabbits given lethal doses systemically. It can act on the ciliary ganglion if injected into the posterior orbit. It does not affect the intrinsic contraction of cardiac muscle. Cats and carion eaters are relatively insensitive to the toxin. The intermediate mechanisms of its action are not known, but it may affect the transport of calcium. Doubling the calcium concentration in tissue temporarily restores neuromuscular conduction after it has been lost due to the action of Botox. Guanidine (4-amino pyridine) can improve muscle strength in humans with clinical botulism.

The toxin can be absorbed orally and is activated by proteolytic nicking and broken down to the 150,000 d size in the intestine by the action of proteases and trypsin. Activation increases the toxicity by a factor greater than 10. Following oral ingestion in humans, extreme variability of systemic effects has been noted. The typical incubation period is 18 hours to several days. The LD_{50} is determined for each batch produced. Each of the currently distributed 100-unit vials contains approximately 25 ng of toxin. The effects of systemic toxicity include gastrointestinal dysfunction, cranial nerve palsies including pupillary and accommodation problems, autonomic difficulties including dry eyes and mouth, and ascending paralysis that impairs walking and respiration [7]. After oral ingestion, intraocular and extraocular muscle paralysis can last as long as 9 months. The reasons for the long duration of action are not understood but two theories are that (1) the toxin may contain amino acid sequences that are not readily degraded by the target tissue, or (2) the toxin attacks a substrate that is only slowly replaced within the motor nerves.

The physiological action of Botox on extraocular muscles may be different and more permanent than on skeletal muscles, such as the orbicularis oculi. Extraocular muscles have a unique and complex fiber-type pattern of which the singly innervated muscle fibers of the orbital layer sustain the most permanent injury following Botox injection. Fibers of this layer are of the "slow" type in that they are rich in mitochondria and resistant to fatigue. The levator palpebrae superioris is an extraocular muscle that is almost constantly in contraction to maintain the eyelid in an open position [8, 9]. Because the levator may be more susceptible to permanent injury than the orbicularis oculi muscle it is best to avoid inadvertent injection of the levator when treating patients with blepharospasm. Thus we recommend an injection pattern for Botox that is over the inferior tarsus at the medial and lateral ends of the eyelids. Histological studies have shown that Botox injection produces atrophy followed by recovery in skeletal muscles [9, 10]. This pattern is more accelerated in the "slow" muscle fiber types than in "fast" muscle fiber types. The orbicularis oculi is primarily composed of "fast" muscle types or "twitch-type" muscle fibers. Evidence for this conclusion comes from electron microscopy, which shows greater demyelination of nerves leading to neuromuscular junctions of twitch-type muscles than of fibers leading to slow-type muscles. Clinical and histological evidence is lacking with regard to long-term changes in orbicularis oculi muscle strength or structure. Preterminal sprouting of axons just prior to neuromuscular junctions in injected muscles has been reported in patients who have later undergone surgical orbicularis myectomy [11]. Similar results were obtained when Botox was injected into the eyelids of monkeys. Preterminal axonal sprouting was the only long-term effect [9]. Thus, there is no reason to believe that Botox will produce cumulative weakening when repeatedly injected into the eyelids.

■ Weakness Distant to Injection Sites

Although injections in the eyelids can spread to adjacent tissues to cause undesirable effects such as ptosis and diplopia, the greatest risks are those that might produce difficulties with respiration and swallowing. Injections into the tongue for lingual dystonia may be followed by dysphagia and aspiration complicated by pneumonia [2]. Botox injections for anterocollis are associated with dysphagia, whereas injections for retrocollis do not seem to involve the inferior pharyngeal constrictor muscles. Patients with weakness of the pharyngeal constrictors may require a liquid diet or gastric feeding tubes. Worse yet, there is the risk of choking and upper airway obstruction with food, such as a piece of meat. Patients with torticollis of all types may demonstrate neck weakness after injection. Botox has been injected into the external pterygoid for mouth opening spasm, but clinical improvement can be compromised by rhinolalia and nasal regurgitation. Abnormalities produced by Botox injections into the eyelid were demonstrated by single-fiber electromyography studies of sites as distant as the lower leg, but these changes were of no clinical significance in these patients [12].

■ Immunology

The immunological aspects of the toxin are being actively studied. The nanogram amounts of the toxin used clinically for treatment of strabismus or eyelid spasms are not usually immunogenic. Each 100 units of the currently licensed product contains approximately 25 ng of protein. The administration of more than 300 units repeated within 30 days may be sufficient to induce antibody production. Scott [1] has reported on 79 patients who were thought to experience limited drug effect; 9 had serum antibodies to type A toxin. Thus, antibody production may complicate treatment of dystonia in large muscles, including torticollis involving the sternocleidomastoid, because doses of 300 units or more may be necessary to achieve the required paralysis. Doses of more than 500 units are likely to render the patient immune to Botox. Ophthalmologists need to be aware of the amount and timing of botulinum toxin being injected into other areas of the body [2]. Several solutions to the problem of needing to limit the dose have been proposed: these include production of a product that contains one-fifth the protein per unit dose of botulinum toxin type A, and use of types B and I botulinum toxin (Alan B. Scott, personal communication).

The biological warfare response to the threat of botulinum toxin type A being placed in a water supply is immunization of the population with a formalin-treated toxoid. Production of a measurable antitoxin antibody titer in humans requires 15 μg of the toxoid. The type A toxin is rapidly removed from the circulating blood, although other types of botulinum toxin may be detected for as long as 25 days. An antitoxin has been produced and it can be used systemically or locally. Systemically, the antitoxin would be of value only if given within approximately 1 hour after exposure to the toxin, because Botox is rapidly absorbed into muscle where it is firmly bound. Local administration of the antitoxin might be of value in containing the effects of the toxin (i.e., giving the antitoxin to one muscle and the toxin to the adjacent muscle). Both the toxin and the antitoxin proteins spread through tissues in approximately the same way, however, so no clinical advantage has yet been demonstrated.

■ Ophthalmic Indications

The ophthalmic indications for the use of Botox relate to the eyelids and to the extraocular muscles. Eyelid conditions amenable to the use of Botox are listed in Table 2.

Extraocular muscle indications for Botox may include early prestabilization treatment of acute abducens nerve paresis or late poststabilization treatment of chronic abducens nerve paresis, where Botox may prevent or release potential medial rectus contracture [13]. Botox can be used as a preoperative or intraoperative medial rectus muscle injection as an adjunct to total transposition of the insertions of the inferior and superior recti in the Jensen procedure for abducens nerve paralysis [14]. Similarly, Botox can be injected into the lateral rectus muscle in cases of oculomotor palsy. Botox is used where surgery is neither desired nor indicated (e.g., eyes likely to have anterior segment necrosis) in the treatment of nonparetic strabismus of less than 20 prism diopters (although deviations of 40 or more prism diopters can be treated, especially if multiple injections are used). Restrictive and endocrine ocular myopathies have also been treated with Botox [15].

A detailed discussion of the dystonic syndromes that may include essential blepharospasm is beyond the scope of this chapter [16]. Table 3 indicates some of the differences between blepharospasm syndromes (a presumed central nervous system neurotransmitter disorder), hemifacial spasm (a facial nerve compressive disorder), and ocular myokymia (a benign condition). Table 4 reviews neurological conditions associated with blepharospasm, and Table 5 lists other ocular conditions that may present as blepharospasm.

Table 2 *Eyelid Indications for Botulinum Toxin*

- I. Orbicularis oculi muscle
  - A. Common blepharospasms
    1. Essential blepharospasm including patients with recurrences following orbicularis myectomy [1, 3, 4, 16, 18, 19, 21, 25, 26]
    2. Hemifacial spasm in patients (alternative or supplement to intracranial neurosurgical microvascular decompression of the facial nerve)
  - B. Other blepharospasms
    1. Acute spastic entropion (usual treatments are everting [Quickert] sutures or adhesive tape)
    2. Senile entropion if inoperable [26]
    3. Pharmacological blepharospasm (including that caused by levodopa used to treat Parkinson's disease and tardative dystonia caused by neuroleptic drugs)
    4. Tourette's syndrome and other facial tics
    5. Progressive supranuclear palsy and Parkinson's disease
    6. Misregeneration of facial nerve (blink associated with smile [27])
- II. Frontalis muscle for apraxia of eyelid opening [22]
- III. Levator palpebrae superioris muscle (indications not yet defined)
  - A. Chemical tarsorrhaphy or protective ptosis (superior rectus weakening will occur in 80%)
    1. Facial nerve palsy with inability to close lids
    2. Indolent corneal ulcers
  - B. Levator retraction resulting from Graves' disease

Table 3 *Differentiating Blepharospasm Syndromes, Hemifacial Spasm, and Ocular Myokymia*

- Blepharospasm
  - Definition: bilateral, simultaneous squeezing of the eyelids
  - Complications include loss of vision when driving and deformities, including brow ptosis, dermatocholasis, disinsertion of the levator aponeurosis, and lateral canthal tendon laxity
  - Most frequently occurs in older women
  - Younger patients are more likely to be "psychogenic"
  - Can be form fruste of dystonia musculorum deformans or a finding in postencephalitic Parkinsonism
  - Absent during sleep
- Meige syndrome (blepharospasm with oromandibular dystonia)
  - Spontaneous or drug induced
  - Dopaminergic hypersensitivity may occur during or upon withdrawal from the postsynaptic blockade caused by dopamine antagonists (neuroleptics)
  - Drug responses similar to those seen in Huntington's disease with dopaminergic preponderance
  - May be preceded by typical tardative dyskinesia
  - May be preceded by drug-induced parkinsonism, akasthisia (restlessness), or dystonia
- Hemifacial spasm
  - Unilateral twitching usually beginning in inferior orbicularis oculi and spreading to corner of mouth, mentalis muscle, and later to the platysma
  - Frontalis involved in only 15%
  - Present during sleep as well as when patient is awake
  - Increased spasm with voluntary and emotional facial movements
  - Tensor tympaini spasm with clicking sound occurs during sleep and can awaken patient from sleep
  - Tonus phenomenon is helpful in diagnosis and a sustained contraction can often be evoked by forced lid closure
  - Head position may modify symptoms
  - Weakness is mild but progressive
  - Patient cannot bury eyelashes, kiss, or whistle
  - Typical hemifacial spasm is caused by cross-compression by a vessel at the anterior caudal aspect of facial nerve root entry zone (REZ)
  - Atypical hemifacial spasm begins in buccal muscles and spreads upward; usually caused by a vessel at the posterior rostral aspect of REZ
  - Median age at onset: 50–60 years
  - Sex: 2F:1M
  - Diagnostic imaging: contrast-enhanced magnetic resonance imaging or computed tomography scan [21] of posterior fossa to rule out tumor (<1%) [28]
  - Operative findings: 95% arterial compression; remaining 5% include mixed arterial and venous compression, compression by tumors
- Ocular myokymia
  - Unilateral twitching
  - Occurs when the patient is awake but the face is at rest
  - No obvious local cause
  - Benign course and resolution

Table 4 *Neurological Conditions Associated with Blepharospasm*[a]

Focal cortical seizures
Apraxia of lid opening occurs in parkinsonism, progressive supranuclear palsy, and Huntington's chorea
Progressive supranuclear palsy
Senile chorea
Athetosis of facial muscles
Wilson's disease
Tourette's syndrome
Facial myokymia of multiple sclerosis or brain stem glioma: undulating, flickering movements of adjacent muscle bundles instead of repeated movements of same muscle bundles
Gaze-evoked orbicularis clonus (sometimes associated with multiple sclerosis)
Aberrant facial nerve regeneration
Myotonias
Dystrophica
Congenita
Chondrodystrophica
Schwartz-Jampel syndrome: blepharospasm, blepharophimosis, facial and skeletal abnormalities
Tetanus
Myasthenia gravis and other causes of binocular diplopia (autosomal recessive myasthenia gravis may present with lid twitching)

[a]From [16].

■ Contraindications

Because eyelid muscles represent relatively easy targets, most patients will be able to cooperate sufficiently for safe injection. This is in contrast to injection into deeper muscles, during which patients must be able to cooperate or be given sedation for insertion of the electromyograph (EMG)-guided needles into a specific muscle. Nevertheless, there may be patients whose globes could be at risk if they cannot remain steady at the time of injection. Local conditions that may represent relative contraindications to injection include preexisting eyelid and brow ptosis, excessive dermatochalasis of the eyelids, or a local infection at the time of a scheduled injection. Relative contraindications of a systemic nature may include bleeding disorders, including recent aspirin use, myasthenia gravis, or the Eaton-Lambert syndrome. The adverse effects of aminoglycoside antibiotics have exacerbated the effects of systemic botulism, but this probably should not be an issue with the Botox doses used in treating systemic blepharospasm. The effects of botulinum toxin on pregnancy are

Table 5 *Ocular Causes of Blepharospasm*

Irritative lesions such as keratitis sicca
Xeroderma pigmentosa
Intraocular lenses
Congenital horizontal tarsal kink syndrome
Relief of monocular diplopia

unknown, but several women have been injected in the first trimester and no known complications have occurred. A history of botulism is not a contraindication to Botox, and patients with demonstrated antibodies to botulinum toxin have not had anaphylaxis or allergic manifestations when challenged with Botox.

■ Overdosage

Systemic complications of overdosage with Botox have thankfully not yet been reported, but some guidance may be obtained from a case of descending paralysis (ophthalmoparesis, bulbar palsy, and limb weakness) that occurred as a result of a subcutaneous cyst infected by botulism in a cocaine abuser [17]. The patient had normal cerebrospinal fluid cell count and chemical profile, responded to edrophonium, and demonstrated weak action potentials on EMG that could be potentiated with repeated stimuli. Pyridostigmine bromide and repeated plasmapheresis treatments led to resolution of the problem after the obscure cyst was located, cultured, and excised. Only 20% of patients with wound botulism have detectable toxin in their serum, but all have abnormal electrophysiological studies.

■ Dosage

Each vial of toxin contains 100 units or approximately 25 ng botulinum type A neurotoxin humagglutinin complex and 0.5 mg human serum albumin to stabilize the drug. The safety, sterility, and potency of the drug are supervised by the FDA on a batch approval basis. The available botulinum toxin type A is stable for years if kept frozen below −5°C. The powder is rediluted with unpreserved 0.9% sterile saline. The solution is diluted to 5 or 10 units per 0.1 ml and drawn up into a tuberculin syringe. We prefer the weaker dilution to control waste; it is sometimes difficult to manage leakage through the rubber stopper around the needle and it is also difficult to get the last drop out of the vial. The threshold dose for extraocular muscle paralysis is 0.3 to 1.5 units. This dosage approximates the amount of toxin that, if spread away from an injection site in the eyelids and into the levator palpebrae superioris or inferior oblique muscles, would result in ptosis or diplopia. The mouse LD_{50} is 0.4 ng. Doses 26 times the mouse LD_{50} have been given to humans without systemic complications.

■ Administration into the Eyelids

Eyelids should be clean and free of cosmetics that might inadvertently be tatooed into the eyelid and give rise to local tissue reactions. A half-inch 30-gauge needle is placed on a 1 ml tuberculin syringe, after a 27-gauge needle supplied with the syringe is used for penetrating the rubber stopper of the Botox vial. Sites of injection in the eyelids are individualized for each patient. Injections may be imprecise with regard to the actual initial distribution of

	FORCE (0–4)	BOTOX UNITS
CORRUGATOR		
BROW		
UPPER LID/PRESEPTAL		
UPPER LID/PRETARSAL	4	10
CANTHUS		5
LOWER LID/PRETARSAL	4	10
LOWER LID/PRESEPTAL		
CHEEK		
ZYGOMATICUS MAJOR		

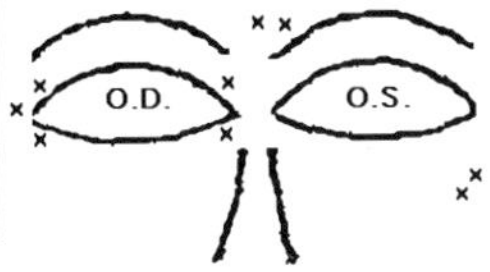

	FORCE (0–4)	BOTOX UNITS
CORRUGATOR	4	10
BROW		
UPPER LID/PRESEPTAL		
UPPER LID/PRETARSAL	1	
CANTHUS		
LOWER LID/PRETARSAL	0	
LOWER LID/PRESEPTAL		
CHEEK	4	10
ZYGOMATICUS MAJOR		

Diagram used to record each injection includes tables for the right and left sides of the face and lists the muscles injected, their force at the time of injection, and the dose of Botulinum toxin (BOTOX) *injected. Usually we record only the force (strength) of the upper and lower eyelids. The "x" marks each injection site and typically indicates 5 units. (Right) The starting injection record for a typical patient is shown. (Left) The record for a hypothetical patient returning for initial follow-up at 1 month. The eyelids are weaker but the patient is still bothered by other muscles, which are injected at this visit.*

solution in the eyelid tissue. There is variation in the back pressure exerted by the tissue and the flow of the injected material through tissue planes. Sometimes a 0.1-ml injection will pool around the tip of the needle, whereas a seemingly identical technique in the contralateral lid will result in fluid 10 mm or more from the needle tip. We have found it convenient to use a rubber stamp to print a diagram of each patient's face on their chart (Figure). The diagram is surrounded on the right and left sides by tables that list the regions of the face and provides spaces that may be used to record severity of spasm symptoms, strength of muscles, and administered dose for each region. The exact location of each injection in each region is marked with an X (usually representing 5 units). Larger or smaller doses are shown by multiples or fractions (e.g., 2X or X/2). Unusual movements of solution away from the needle site or the location of significant bruises can be marked. A simple notation can be used to indicate distance in mm from the eyelid margin if it is significant. One patient for whom these notations have been useful had a facelift prior to developing blepharospasm. The facial nerve supply to her perioral region may have been shifted upward near the zygomatic arch so we avoided recurrent undesired weakness by keeping the injections close to the eyelid. Many older patients develop lower eyelid weakness when the injection is close to the lower eyelid ectropion margin, so the injection should be moved 10 mm or more below the eyelid margin. Some patients with hemifacial spasm have opposing cocontraction of their frontalis and orbicularis oculi muscles during their spasms. In these patients it is important to observe that the frontalis contraction tends to raise the eyebrow and to elevate the eyelid. In such cases, the nerve supply to the frontalis muscle should be protected from the Botox injection. The examiner should be alert to identify this phenomenon and to avoid injections more than 3 cm lateral to the orbital rim, thus protecting the branches of the facial nerve.

The anatomical basis for the efficacy of Botox in treating blepharospasm is not completely known. We have determined that the pretarsal portion of the orbicularis oculi muscle in rabbits and monkeys contains almost all type II (twitch) fibers, whereas the preseptal portions of the muscle are composed of an increasing proportion of type I (slow) fibers. The slow fibers are those that can sustain continuous, forceful contraction because their energy is directly derived from oxidative metabolism involving mitochondria, whereas the twitch fibers depend on glycogen. Moreover, the muscle fiber diameters of both fiber types increase as a function of distance from the eyelid margin. If these observations can be extended to humans, then the resting tone of the pretarsal portion of the eyelids may not require muscle discharge, at least when patients are awake. Ocular closure during sleep might depend on continuous contraction of the type I fibers. Contraction of these relatively weak pretarsal twitch fibers is the initiating event of eyelid closure followed by recruitment of both larger type II and slower type I contracting fibers as the eyelids close more tightly. We are not certain that patients will experience sufficient relief from blepharospasms if only the preseptal and orbital (more peripheral) portions of the muscle are paralyzed. Elston [18, 19] in Great Britain, however, uses an injection pattern of 1 ng (approximately 4 units in the United States) in the lateral aspect, and 0.5 ng in the medial aspect of the upper lid, just below the eyebrow, and in the lower lid at its lateral and central portions similar distances from the eyelid margin. His rationale is that the orbital portion of the orbicularis is responsible for forceful closure of the eyelids and that gentle closure should be preserved. He claims that this method limits complications such as ptosis and diplopia. He reports, however, that ptosis sufficient to obstruct vision and diplopia occurred in 4.8% of cases [16, 17]. This percentage is nearly equivalent to results reported by American investigators who generally inject much closer to, if not at, the eyelid margins. Studies of patients with lid spasms injected with Botox show that the levator palpebrae muscle relaxes during a downward lid saccade and that contraction of the orbicularis oculi muscle does not have an important role in this movement [20]. Botox-induced weakening of the orbicularis oculi decreased both the amplitude and the peak velocity of the blink downphase, indicating a role for the orbicularis in the physiology of normal blinking.

American investigators tend to inject the toxin into the medial and lateral pretarsal regions of the upper eyelids and the lateral pretarsal portion of the lower eyelids (claiming that this avoids lower eyelid ectropion). Frueh and Musch [21] claim that lower eyelid injections for blepharospasm are generally unnecessary, but we think this claim is overstated. One basis for their statement is that some patients with blepharospasm obtain significant relief from myectomy of the upper eyelid protractors. They also point out that lower lid injections frequently lead to inferior oblique muscle paresis and diplopia. We agree with both of these assertions and note that lower eyelid injection alone will not satisfy any patient except those whose hemifacial spasm involves only the lower eyelids. We usually inject the medial portion of the lower eyelids as well. To our knowledge, treatment in the lateral aspect of the orbicularis has not been systematically investigated because it has been the custom to follow Scott and assign each dose to the upper and lower eyelid. Nevertheless, we frequently inject the lateral canthal region particularly as a way to avoid upper eyelid injections in patients whose local eyelid tissue seems to predispose them to ptosis. We have previously mentioned an exception to extreme lateral injections when there is frontalis cocontraction in hemifacial spasm.

The package circular accompanying Oculinum recommends starting doses of one-quarter to one-half those suggested here. Our typical starting doses for patients without preexisting eyelid or brow ptosis are 5 units at the most medial and lateral aspects of the upper eyelid close to the lash line, 5 units 1 cm lateral to the lateral canthus, and 5 units medially and laterally in the preseptal portion of the lower eyelid. This produces an initial starting dose of 25 units per eye, possibly supplemented by 5 units in the procerus/corrugator region of each side of the face. We decrease the initial dose if there are eyelid problems or a history of prior orbicularis myectomy [19]. The range of repeated treatment doses for an eyelid is between 5 and 35 units per eyelid; this total is increased if the procerus, the orbital portions of the orbicularis oculi, the cheek, the zygomaticus major, or the buccinator muscles are further treated (dose can equal 50 units per eye). In patients with hemifacial spasm, the dose on one side of the face may be further increased by injecting unit amounts of Botox into the levator labii superioris and orbicularis oris muscles and 5 units into the mentalis muscles. To prevent drooling and other symptoms that patients fear will not subside, we defer such injections to the initial follow-up or subsequent scheduled injections, after which patients will better understand the effects of drug action.

■ Instructions Given to Patients

Patients are usually told to stop or taper drugs that have been prescribed but seem ineffective in controlling spasms. After each injection, patients are routinely prescribed a sterile ophthalmic lubricating ointment and are told to start using it the second or third night after injection when lower eyelid weakness or even ectropion may appear. This ointment prevents drying of the inferior cornea during sleep. We tell patients to continue using the ointment until they are certain that they are not having dry eye symptoms or until it begins to be difficult to instill the ointment due to increased lower eyelid strength. Patients are instructed to call if there is blurring of vision beyond that expected from the ointment or if there is pain that suggests a corneal abrasion or ulcer. We warn patients that they may develop unwanted ptosis (occurs in approximately 11% of injections, some of which will be bilateral and cause obstruction of vision) or weakness of other ocular muscles beginning as late as several weeks after orbital injection. Paralytic ectropion can contribute to corneal dryness with irritation and excessive reflex tearing that occur in approximately 10% of injections. Tearing symptoms may also result from weakening of the lacrimal sac pump mechanism. Keratitis and even corneal ulcers may occur following eyelid injections. Entropion has been reported, but we have never seen it following injection. These adverse effects generally recede as the muscles regain their strength. We reassure patients concerning mild amounts of ptosis or diplopia. Adhesive tape may help with bilateral ptosis. Patients are told to patch one eye if diplopia is causing spatial disorientation. We also tell patients that eyelid edema or rash may occur and that in rare instances there may be a flu-like syndrome with generalized weakness and nausea. If such symptoms occur they are most likely due to something else. To limit hematomas at the injection sites we ask patients to refrain, if possible, from the use of aspirin for 2 weeks before and from the use of nonsteroidal antiinflammatory agents for 2 days before the next scheduled Botox injection.

■ Postinjection Follow-up and Readministration

We attempt to see each patient approximately 1 month after the initial administration of Botox. This schedule gives us the opportunity to see the peak effect of the initial dose and any side effects. We can reassure patients concerning ptosis and diplopia and evaluate lower eyelid weakness or malposition as well as midfacial weakness. These observations will allow adjustment of the amount and placement of subsequent doses. We try to wait at least 3 months for the next injection so patients learn about the effectiveness of the treatment cycle. Many patients will find there are times they can go up to 4 or 5 months between injections because of unexplained fluctuation in their symptoms. Sometimes additional sites are treated at the initial 1-month return visit. These sites are usually the procerus and corrugator muscles in patients with essential blepharospasm or the zygomaticus major muscle in patients with hemifacial spasm.

The initial follow-up visit is important from a psychological and adjunctive therapy standpoint. Some patients have settled into a less social life-style because the spasms become an excuse for dependency and isolation. It is important to demonstrate that the spasms are really absent or substantially improved. They may need to be encouraged to return to driving and performing errands for themselves. They may need encouragement to get more involved socially.

The initial follow-up visit also provides an opportunity to change, increase, or decrease dosages of drugs such as lorazepam or carbamazepine. This follow-up visit also allows an evaluation as to whether the patient should receive further injections or be referred for injection at other sites of focal dystonia. The initial follow-up examination may also confirm the impression that injection alone will not be sufficient treatment for the eyelids due to structural problems and that the patient will require oculoplastic surgery to correct problems such as brow or eyelid ptosis, dermatochalasis, lateral canthal disinsertion, or lower eyelid laxity.

Later follow-up visits are primarily used for reinjection. It is recommended that no more than 300 units of Botox be administered in a 3-month period. In our experience, some patients with severe dystonia require injections at 2-month intervals. Larger doses are used if injection is required more frequently than every 3 months, but a point is reached at which no further improvement occurs and the increased dosage is often accompanied by unwanted ptosis and ectropion.

■ Apparent Change of Diagnosis

Our experience following eyelid Botox injections is that there is a decrease in the number of prior diagnoses and increased recognition of misdiagnosis. Sometimes we become aware of incomplete diagnosis. Most of our patients have been treated for dry eye syndromes and many have been considered to have functional psychogenic disorders. Certainly some of these patients have dry eyes and demonstrated a tear production deficiency on Schirmer filter paper strip testing. After Botox treatment, however, many of these patients experience a significant reduction in their use of lubricant drops and ointments. Behavior patterns of many treated patients normalizes and their previously "neurotic" symptoms disappear. Some patients with essential blepharospasm have relatively unilateral onset and these patients may be injected unilaterally on the first visit because they believe that the opposite eye is squeezing in "sympathy." At the follow-up visit it is clear that the uninjected side is involved also. We have never seen bilateral hemifacial spasm (with independent timing of contraction on the opposite side of the face). Tumors are a rare cause of hemifacial spasm [21]. When correctly diagnosed, patients with hemifacial spasm who reappear with blinking of the opposite eye will do so because of corneal irritation of the treated eye. We have also recognized apraxia of eyelid opening, which can coexist with or be independent of blepharospasm [22]. This diagnosis is of course more easily made if the eyelid cannot be voluntarily opened or when the eyelid can no longer be squeezed shut following Botox treatment for presumed blepharospasm. The normal function of the levator can be confirmed by the doll's head maneuver or by startling the patient and then asking them to open their eyes.

■ Botox Results

Evaluation of eyelid (and other) spasms is largely subjective on the part of each patient, each patient's family, and treating physicians. Various closed trials have sought to overcome bias through videotape examinations scored by independent observers. We believe that open trials are best for Botox treatment because patients and physicians can adjust the dosage site and amount on the basis of the reported experience. More than 90% of patients experience substantial improvement within 1 to 5 days after injection. Most patients score their spasms as debilitating or nearly so prior to Botox injection and change to absent to mild after injection. The average duration of satisfactory response is 13 weeks, approximately 7% of patients claim the effects last less than 4 weeks. These patients may seek surgery or even disability status. Approximately 6% of patients claim improvement lasting up to 6 months. Most of these patients have hemifacial spasm and may be more tolerant because their condition is unilateral, but some are patients with blepharospasm, which can go into periods of remission. The temporary paralysis caused by the injection is not demonstrable for longer than 4 to 5 months. Botox has offered dramatic relief to patients who previously had little or no response to pharmacological therapy or only a temporary response to orbicularis myectomy or facial nerve microvascular decompression. The main criticism of Botox therapy is its temporary nature and cost in patient time and in medical resources.

■ Alternative Treatments

Pharmacological Agents

A review of the pharmacological agents used for treatment of dystonias is beyond the scope of this review. In general, these drugs modify, enhance, or decrease central neurotransmitter function. Botox has made them largely adjunctive agents for eyelid spasms, but many ophthalmology patients have mild to severe aspects of orofacial dystonia that need attention. Treating these problems may lead to an improvement in the blepharospasm symptoms. These drugs include anticholinergics, baclofen, benzodiazepines, dopamine depleters, and lithium.

Orbicularis Myectomy

Before the introduction of orbicularis myectomy by Gillum and Anderson in 1981, surgical treatment for eyelid spasms was differential section of the facial nerve [16]. The nerve section had an unsatisfactory rate of immediate success and the long-term failure rate was even worse. Jordan and colleagues [16] continue to revise the orbicularis myectomy and it has an acceptable level of long-term success. It also provides a surgical approach to deal with anatomical deformities that result from or complicate the treatment of blepharospasm. The procedure carries with it the cost of several hours of general anesthesia and one or more nights in the hospital due to the need to evacuate hematomas and treat lid edema and ecchymosis. Full healing may take up to 1 year. Touch-up procedures or later reoperation may be necessary to control recurrent spasms or other problems. We have successfully used Botox in patients who were not free of spasm following orbicularis myectomy. It is our impression that the operation and the Botox injections are complimentary.

Chemomyectomy

Our group has been engaged in a still-experimental effort to develop a more permanent treatment for eyelid and other spasms. We have investigated the use of intramuscular injections of doxorubicin preceded by a mixture of bupivacaine hydrochloride, epinephrine, and hyaluronidase. To prevent development of a major ulcer of the eyelid, the dose of doxorubicin must be limited. With our present protocol we suspect that as many as 3 injections may be necessary in each treated region [23]. Each injection is followed by swelling and tenderness. The degree of weakness is not as great as produced by Botox. Nevertheless, cumulative muscle weakness and decreased spasm result, and a clinical trial is in progress. We are investigating other cotreatments that will amplify the destructive effects on the orbicularis muscle while minimizing damage to the eyelid skin. Chemomyectomy is not the only pharmacological approach to obtaining a longer lasting result. It has been proposed to use agents that may delay or prevent sprouting of preterminal axons that may contribute to the functional recovery of muscle paralyzed with Botox.

■ Comments

Botulinum toxin type A has been established as a safe and effective temporary treatment for essential blepharospasm and hemifacial spasm. It also appears to be useful in other neurological disorders, and the list of conditions for which it is used is continuing to expand. Moreover, the success of this therapy has led to the recognition that muscle spasms need not be tolerated, and that additional therapeutic approaches need to be developed. Current research with other types and formulations of botulinum toxin may give relief to those patients who have become immune to the effects of botulinum type A. Surgical orbicularis myectomy will continue to play an important role in the treatment of these patients, and chemomyectomy appears to be a promising approach. The management of spasm is no longer a static field of endeavor.

■ References

1. Scott AB, Kennedy RA, Stubbs HA. Botulinum A toxin injection as a treatment for blepharospasm. Arch Ophthalmol 1986;103:347–350
2. Clinical use of botulinum toxin. (Reprinted from NIH Consens Dev Conf Consens Statement, 1990 Nov 12–14;8[8].)
3. American Academy of Neurology. Assessment: the clinical usefulness of Botulinum toxin-A in treating neurological disorders. Neurology 1990;40:1332–1336
4. American Academy of Ophthalmology. Botulinum toxin therapy of eye muscle disorders: safety and effectiveness. Ophthalmology 1989;96(suppl):37–41
5. Simpson LL. Molecular pharmacology of botulinum toxin and tetanus toxin. Ann Rev Pharmacol Toxicol 1986;26:427–453
6. Smith LD. Botulism: the organism, its toxin, the disease. Springfield: CC Thomas, 1977
7. Folberg JW, Trobe JD. Botulism. In Gold DH, Weingeist TA, eds. The eye in systemic disease. Philadelphia: JB Lippincott, 1990:157–159
8. Porter JD, Burns LA, May PJ. Morphological substrate for eyelid movements: innervation and structure of primate levator palpebrae superioris and orbicularis oculi muscles. J Comp Neurol 1989;287:64–81
9. Porter JD, Stebeck S, Capra NF. Botulinum-induced changes in monkey eyelid muscle: comparison with changes seen in extraocular muscle. Arch Ophthalmol 1991;109:396–404
10. Harris CP, Alderson K, Nebeker J, et al. Histological features of human orbicularis oculi treated with Botulinum A toxin. Arch Ophthalmol 1991;109:393–395
11. Holds JB, Alderson K, Fogg SG, Anderson RL. Motor nerve sprouting in human orbicularis oculi after Botulinum A injection. Invest Ophthalmol Vis Sci 1990; 31:178–181
12. Sanders DB, Massey EW, Buckley EG. Botulinum toxin for blepharospasm: single-fiber EMG studies. Neurology 1986;36:545–547
13. Kraft SP, Allan O. The use of Botulinum toxin in the management of abducens nerve palsy. Am Orthop J 1989;39:89–97
14. Rosenbaum AL, Kushner BJ, Kirshen DL. Vertical rectus muscle transposition and botulinum toxin to medial rectus for abducens palsy. Arch Ophthalmol 1989; 107:820–823
15. Dunn WJ, Arnold AC, O'Connor PS. Botulinum toxin for the treatment of dysthyroid ocular myopathy. Ophthalmology 1986;93:470–475
16. Jordan DR, Patrinely JR, Anderson RL, Thiese SM. Essential blepharospasm and related dystonias. Surv Ophthalmol 1989;34:123–132
17. Rapoport MD, Watkins PB. Descending paralysis resulting from acute wound botulism. Ann Neurol 1984;16:359–361
18. Elston JS. Long-term results of treatment of idiopathic blepharospasm with Botulinum toxin injections. Br J Ophthalmol 1987;71:664–668
19. Elston JS, Russell RW. Effect of treatment with Botulinum toxin on neurogenic blepharospasm. Br J Med Clin Res 1985;290:1857–1859

20. Manning KA, Evinger C, Sibony PA. Eyelid movements before and after Botulinum therapy in patients with eyelid spasm. Ann Neurol 1990;28:653–660
21. Frueh BR, Musch DC. Treatment of facial spasm with Botulinum toxin: an interim report. Ophthalmology 1986;93:917–923
22. Katz B, Rosenberg JH. Botulinum therapy for apraxia of lid opening. Am J Ophthalmol 1985;100:305–307
23. Wirtschafter JD. Clinical doxorubicin chemomyectomy: an experimental treatment for eyelid spasms. Ophthalmology 1991;98:357–366
24. Ludlow CL. Treatment of speech and voice disorders with Botulinum toxin. JAMA 1990;264:2671–2675
25. Carruthers J, Stubbs HA. Botulinum toxin for benign essential blepharospasm, hemifacial spasm, and age-related lower eyelid entropion. Can J Neurol Sci 1987;14:42–45
26. Engstrom PF, Arnoult JV, Mazow ML, et al. Effectiveness of Botulinum toxin in the treatment of blepharospasm. Ophthalmology 1987;94:971–975
27. Putterman AM. Botulinum toxin injections in the treatment of seventh nerve misdirection. Am J Ophthalmol 1990;110:205–206
28. Sprick C, Wirtschafter JD. Hemifacial spasm due to intracranial tumor: an international survey of botulinum toxin investigators. Ophthalmology 1988;95:1042–1045

Neuro-ophthalmology: Odds and Ends

Lanning B. Kline, M.D.

Although this edition of *International Ophthalmology Clinics* is not meant to be a comprehensive review of neuro-ophthalmology, there are some important topics not yet discussed. First, I would like to briefly discuss material of particular interest to general ophthalmologists. Dr J. L. Smith would describe these as "neuro-ophthalmological pearls." Second, there are two subjects worthy of more comprehensive review: the molecular genetics of Leber's hereditary optic neuropathy, and traumatic optic neuropathy. I would like to thank Drs Volpe and Lessell for their contributions in discussing the latter topic.

Nine Neuro-ophthalmological "Pearls"

1. Dural Cavernous Fistula

Often exacerbations of signs and symptoms of dural cavernous arteriovenous malformations indicate increased blood flow through the fistula, and strong consideration should be given for some type of endovascular therapy. Sergott and colleagues [1] described three patients with spontaneous dural cavernous fistulas who had marked worsening of their neuro-ophthalmological signs and subsequent complete resolution of symptoms. Cerebral angiography in all three patients and magnetic resonance imaging (MRI) in two demonstrated thrombosis of the entire superior ophthalmic vein. All patients subsequently underwent spontaneous, complete resolution of symptoms. The value of MRI is underscored in evaluating patients with dural cavernous fistula who experience apparent worsening of their clinical findings. Indeed, they may require no additional treatments and appear to have an excellent prognosis.

2. Acquired Immunodeficiency Syndrome (AIDS)

The ophthalmologic manifestations of human immunodeficiency virus (HIV) infection are protean. Virtually every portion of the central nervous system may be affected, leading to an almost limitless range of neuro-ophthalmological findings. Conditions such as tuberculosis and syphilis, thought to be very rare just a few years ago, now must be considered in the appropriate patient population presenting with visual loss, visual field defects,

Table 1 *Neuro-ophthalmic Findings in AIDS—Literature Review*

Cranial nerve palsies
CNS infections (toxoplasmosis, cryptococcosis, varicella zoster, PML, CMV)
CNS lymphoma (primary or metastatic)
Orbital lymphoma
Cavernous and orbital apex eosinophilic granuloma
Optic neuropathy
Papilledema (cryptococcal meningitis, CNS toxoplasmosis, CNS lymphoma)
Optic neuritis (CMV, syphilitic, varicella zoster, hepatitis B, toxoplasmic)
Retrobulbar optic neuritis (syphilitic, CMV, cryptococcal)
Optic nerve perineuritis (syphilitic, cryptococcal)
Anterior ischemic optic neuropathy
Toxic optic neuropathy (e.g., ethambutol toxicity)
Optic atrophy as a sequelae of the neuropathy
Eye movement disorders
Slowed saccades and abnormal optokinetic response (HIV encephalopathy, CMV encephalitis)
Progressive convergence insufficiency
Reverse ocular dipping (cryptococcal meningitis)
Parinaud's syndrome (herpes encephalitis, HIV encephalopathy)
Internuclear ophthalmoplegia (CMV encephalitis, cerebral mucormycosis)
PPRF lesions (HIV encephalopathy)
Blepharospasm (HIV encephalopathy)
Opsoclonus
Skew deviation
Visual field defects
Homonymous hemianopsia (PML, cryptococcal meningitis, internal carotid occlusion from meningovascular syphilis)
Homonymous quadrantanopsia (CNS astrocytoma)
Enlarged blind spot (PML)
Pericentral scotoma (PML)
Miscellaneous
Cortical blindness (cryptococcal meningitis, CNS tuberculosis)
Visual allesthesia
Visual hallucination
Photophobia (cryptococcal meningitis)

AIDS = acquired immunodeficiency syndrome; CNS = central nervous system; PML = progressive multifocal leukoencephalopathy; CMV = cytomegalovirus; HIV = human immunodeficiency virus; PPRF = pontine paramedian reticular formation.

From [3]. Used with permission.

and abnormal eye movements. This is underscored by the report of Winward and associates [2], who described four patients (three men, one woman) all in the third and fourth decades of life who had optic nerve dysfunction. Although the most likely diagnosis of patients in this age range would be idiopathic or demyelinative optic neuritis, these four patients, all of whom were HIV-positive, had diverse causes for their optic neuropathy: syphilitic optic perineuritis, cytomegalovirus papillitis, varicella zoster optic neuritis, and cryptococcal retrobulbar neuritis. Mansour [3] tabulated the spectrum of neuro-ophthalmological complications in AIDS (Table 1).

3. Pharmacological Pupillary Testing for Horner's Syndrome

Kardon and co-workers [4] found topical 10% cocaine drops highly effective in separating normal subjects from patients with Horner's syndrome. Measuring the postcocaine anisocoria provided a better prediction of Horner's syndrome than taking the trouble to calculate the net change in anisooria. The authors provided a table giving the odds of the patient having Horner's syndrome by knowing the final anisocoria value. In a similar fashion, another report [5] from the same institution studied the effects of 1% hydroxyamphetamine hydrobromide (Paredrine, Smith Kline and French Laboratories, Philadelphia, PA) in distinguishing preganglionic from postganglionic lesions in patients with Horner's syndrome. This pharmacological agent was found to be very helpful in making this important clinical distinction. Once again, a table gives the probability that a lesion is postganglionic depending on the difference in pupillary dilation to Paredrine.

4. Spontaneous Internal Carotid Artery Dissection

Dissection of the craniocerebral arteries is an important cause of cerebrovascular symptoms, especially in young adults. Major neurological complications include transient ischemic attack and stroke, but a variety of other symptoms have been reported, including light-headedness, pulsatile tinnitus, lingual paresis, dysgeusia, scalp tenderness, facial numbness, and swelling in the neck [6–8]. Ophthalmological involvement also frequently occurs, yet has only recently been emphasized in the literature [9]. Reported involvement includes postganglionic Horner's syndrome, transient monocular blindness, homonymous visual field defects, ocular ischemic syndrome, and sixth nerve palsy [6, 7, 9–11]. The most frequent ophthalmic complication is transient unilateral blurring or loss of vision, occurring in 6 to 30% of cases. Some of these episodes may be associated with photophobia and scintillations.

Early reports, often based on autopsy studies, associated this disorder with a high mortality rate [12, 13], but recent publications suggest a better prognosis [6, 7]. While carotid angiography has been used to establish the diagnosis, MRI may be a noninvasive method of equal diagnostic accuracy [14]. Because of the uncertainty of the natural history of this condition, a variety of therapeutic approaches, both medical and surgical, have been used. A unified approach to management has yet to appear in the literature.

5. Optic Tract Syndrome

In discussing three patients who sustained optic tract injury after temporal lobectomy, Anderson and colleagues [15] delineated the spectrum of optic tract syndrome. From an anatomical standpoint, distinction is made whether the anterior or posterior optic tract is involved. Table 2 summarizes the major features of each. Type I is actually more frequent than Type II, and is a "junction syndrome" due to a compressive lesion at the junction of the optic nerve, chiasm, and optic tract. This combination results in signs of both optic nerve and optic tract dysfunction. Thus, there is a unilateral reduction in

Table 2 *Optic Tract Syndromes*

	Type I	Type II
Visual acuity	Usually subnormal in ipsilateral eye	Normal
Afferent pupillary defect	Ipsilateral eye	Contralateral eye
Visual field defects	Contralateral complete or incomplete homonymous hemianopia	Contralateral complete or incomplete homonymous hemianopia
Optic disc	Ipsilateral diffuse pallor, contralateral bow-tie pallor	Ipsilateral temporal pallor or normal, contralateral bow-tie pallor
Lesion location	Anterior optic tract and optic nerve	Posterior optic tract
Causes	Mass lesion	Infarction, demyelination, mass lesion

From [15]. Used with permission.

visual acuity with an afferent pupillary defect in that eye. Visual field testing demonstrates a contralateral homonymous hemianopia, and usual causes include tumor and aneurysm. Type II is the traditional optic tract syndrome and occurs very rarely. Acuity is normal in each eye, and the afferent pupillary defect is in the eye with temporal visual field loss. The more posterior portion of the optic tract is involved, usually due to infarction or demyelination.

6. Third Nerve Palsy and the Pupil

In an important editorial, Trobe [16] discusses "footnotes" to the rule of the pupil in third nerve palsy. A series of reports in the 1950s and 1960s led to the following clinical guidelines. If the pupil is involved in a third nerve palsy, the etiology is probably compressive, and potentially life-threatening lesions (e.g., aneurysm) must be excluded. On the other hand, if the pupil is uninvolved ("spared") the probable cause is a microvascular infarction, the likely cause (e.g., diabetes mellitus, hypertension) is benign, and prognosis for recovery is excellent. Trobe [16] emphasizes that this rule is very helpful in clinical decision making provided the following four constraints are heeded:

1. Between the ages of 20 and 50 years, the chances of a compressive lesion, especially aneurysm, is high even if the pupil is spared. Cerebral angiography is indicated in this age group. Below age 20, aneurysms are so rare that angiography can be avoided if there are no clinical signs of subarachnoid hemorrhage and other neuroimaging studies (CT, MRI) are negative.
2. Do not apply the rule when the extraocular palsy is incomplete. If some but not all of the oculomotor-innervated muscles are completely impaired, or if all of the muscles are impaired but only slightly, then pupil sparing may exist with aneurysm.

3. One must be cautious in evaluating patients who have complete oculomotor-innervated extraocular muscle palsy, but only partial iris sphincter palsy or "relative pupil sparing." The literature provides no guidelines as to how often "relative pupil sparing" occurs with aneurysm.
4. Clinicians must be certain that the third nerve palsy is truly isolated (i.e., there are no additional findings from history or physical examination to suspect another cause). For example, a patient with a history of known carcinoma or accompanying neurological signs (e.g., sixth nerve palsy, hemiparesis) would require further evaluation. This exception acknowledges that infarcts and aneurysms are not the only cause of third nerve palsy.

Trobe concludes his editorial warning clinicians: "the rule lives, but mind the footnotes."

7. Optic Disc Drusen and Decreased Visual Acuity

Visual field defects have been reported in 71% of eyes with visible optic disc drusen and in 25 to 39% of eyes with pseudopapilledema but no visible drusen [17, 18]. Reduction in visual acuity, however, is rare. Beck and co-workers [19] reported four patients with visual loss to the point of legal blindness from optic disc drusen. In general, the visual loss occurred in an acute and nonprogressive or step-wise fashion, with visual field loss in a nerve fiber bundle distribution. Visual acuity was not reduced until visual field constriction was severe. The authors caution that reduced acuity from drusen remains a diagnosis of exclusion. All patients should initially undergo cranial CT or MRI. The authors advise caution about declaring drusen as the cause of a central scotoma with only minimal visual field loss. In such cases, the visual loss is probably not related to the drusen, and full evaluation of these patients is warranted to look for another cause of optic neuropathy.

8. Automated Perimetry and Functional Visual Field Loss

Smith and Baker [20] performed visual field testing using an automated static threshold technique in 15 consecutive patients with functional visual field loss. The pattern of abnormality was not distinguishable from organic loss. No form of reliability testing, including number of repetitions, false-positive or false-negative results, root mean square evaluation, or percentage of fixation losses, was capable of characterizing functional deficits. To quote the authors: "Automated perimetry as currently practiced cannot differentiate functional from organic loss. Manual field testing is the procedure of choice in patients with functional visual loss."

9. Ophthalmological Accompaniments of Alzheimer's Disease

Alzheimer's disease is a degenerative neurological disorder characterized by insidious onset of a progressive dementia in middle and late life. It is only within the past few years that the visual disturbances of this disorder have been reported in the ophthalmological literature [21–23]. What these reports may not consistently emphasize is that visual symptoms may be an early manifestation of this disorder. Visual acuity and visual fields are initially normal. The patient often reports reading difficulties at the onset of the disease, but these complaints are usually vague. A variety of other visual deficits may be present, including inability to pick out individual objects from among a group of objects, specific inability to recognize faces, becoming lost in customarily familiar surroundings, and various types of visuospatial disorientation. These individuals live in what has been called a world of "seeing without recognizing." Defects have been quantitated in various objective tests of vision including color vision, spatial contrast sensitivity, fundus examination, ocular motility, higher cortical visual function, visual evoked potential, and pattern electroretinography. Pathological studies in patients with Alzheimer's disease have shown abnormalities at all levels of visual apparatus from retinal ganglion cell to visual cortex.

To date, there is no available therapy for Alzheimer's disease. Yet, ophthalmologists can have an important role in the care of these patients: accurate recognition of visual complaints, prompt referral to allow accurate diagnosis, understanding, and compassion.

■ Leber's Hereditary Optic Neuropathy

The impact of molecular genetics in understanding hereditary metabolic disorders has been felt in virtually every medical specialty. Advances in ophthalmology include isolation of the retinoblastoma gene [24], mapping of the retinitis pigmentosa genes [25], classification of X-linked color vision abnormalities [26], and discovery of the genetic mutation causing gyrate choroidal atrophy [27, 28]. Recently, this technology has been applied to a visually devastating neuro-ophthalmological disorder, Leber's hereditary optic neuropathy (LHON). This brief review illustrates how the field of molecular biology has profoundly altered our understanding of this optic nerve disorder [29–31].

The vast majority of metabolic diseases in which a genetic defect has been found is due to alterations in DNA found within the nucleus of the cell. Recently, a variety of disorders, including LHON, have been shown to be the result of a mutation in the extranuclear mitochondrial DNA (mtDNA). Accounting for approximately 0.3% of the cell's total DNA, the structure and function of mtDNA will be discussed after reviewing the role of the mitochondrion within the cell.

Living organisms need energy, and most is obtained by the breakdown of adenosine triphosphate (ATP) into adenosine diphosphate, inorganic phosphate, and free energy. ATP must be continually produced to meet the demands of the organism. In an average mammalian cell, an ATP molecule will last only one to two minutes. In one day, a resting human produces and uses up to 40 kg of ATP.

Approximately 90% of our ATP is produced by the hundreds of mitochondria within the cytoplasm of each cell. Specifically, ATP is produced by a multimolecular system, the respiratory chain, located in the inner of the two

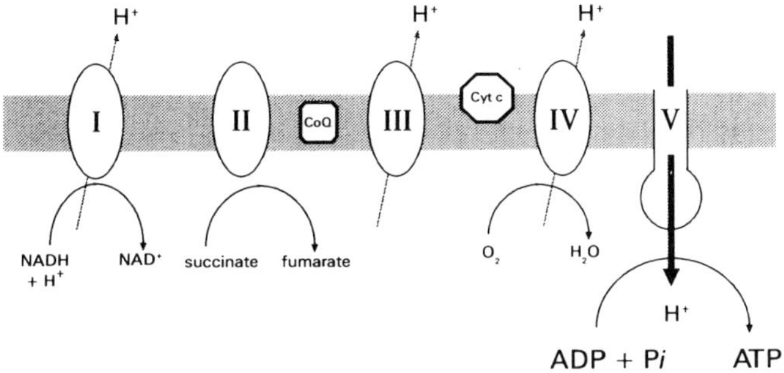

Figure 1 *The major elements of the respiratory chain of the mitochondria. The enzyme complexes are numbered I through V.* CoQ *= coenzyme Q;* Cyt c *= cytochrome c;* ADP *= adenosine diphosphate;* ATP *= adenosine triphosphate. (From [30]. Used with permission.)*

mitochondrial membranes. The chain contains five major complexes of proteins and various prosthetic groups (complexes I–V) and two smaller molecules, coenzyme Q and cytochrome c. In the presence of oxygen, the first four complexes and the two smaller molecules use the energy from our food to generate a proton gradient across the inner mitochondrial membrane. The fifth complex then allows these protons to flow back into the mitochondrion, while harnessing the energy of the gradient to synthesize ATP (Fig 1).

Each mitochondrion contains between two and 20 mtDNA molecules. Like nuclear DNA, mtDNA is read onto messenger RNA, which in turn leads to translation into proteins by ribosomes. The entire process takes place within the mitochondrion.

The human mitochondrial chromosome is a circular molecule of approximately 16,500 base pairs of DNA (Fig 2). It has two complimentary strands of DNA that differ in weight as a result of their chemical composition. They are termed *H (heavy)* and *L (light) strands.* The chromosome carries 37 genes, 13

Figure 2 *Genetic map of the human mitochondrial chromosome. The small circles represent transfer RNA genes. All other genes are identified outside the circle:* ND *=* *NADH dehydrogenase subunits (complex I);* CYB *= cytochrome b subunit (complex III);* CO *= cytochrome c oxidone subunits (complex IV);* ATP *= adenosine triphosphate synthase subunits (complex V). Inside the circle:* O *= origins of replication of heavy* (H) *and light* (L) *strands of the chromosome; and* LHON, *position 11778, the site of the mutation responsible for many cases of Leber's hereditary optic neuropathy. (From [30]. Used with permission.)*

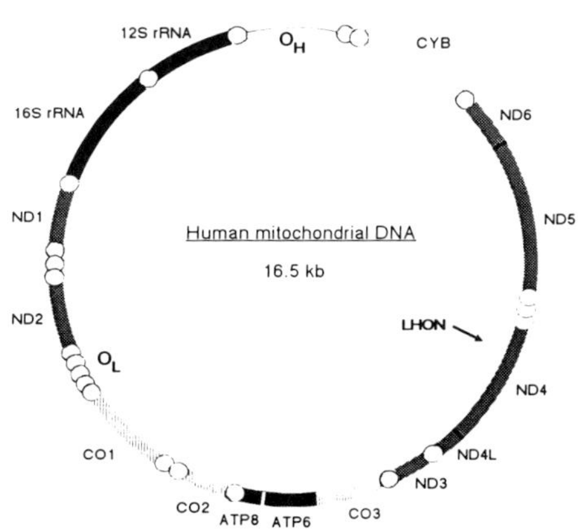

of which encode essential proteins of the respiratory chain, including subunits of complexes I, III, IV, and V. The remaining 24 encode ribosomal and transfer RNA molecules whose sole function is the production of these proteins. Thus, mutations in human mtDNA can lead to diseases caused by deficient energy production.

The inheritance of mtDNA is non-Mendelian. It has been shown in humans as in many other species that an individual receives only maternal mtDNA. During sexual reproduction the cytoplasmic contents (including all mitochondria) are provided by the mother's ovum. The father's sperm cytoplasm is apparently lost. Therefore, offspring inherit only their mother's mtDNA. In addition, mtDNA mutates faster than nuclear DNA. Comparison of the DNA of human and other mammalian mitochondria has shown that the gene sequence changes at least six times more rapidly in mitochondria than in the nucleus.

As mtDNA replicates, the mitochondria divide asymmetrically without regard to mtDNA content or timing of replication. When new mutations occur in mtDNA, there is a period of mixed intracellular population of mutant and normal mtDNA molecules. This condition is termed *heteroplasmy*. At each cellular division of a heteroplasmic cell, the inclusion of mutant and normal mtDNA molecules within the daughter cells is random. Hence, during cellular replication the proportion of mutant and normal mtDNA can drift by a process called replicative segregation. Because mtDNA encodes only energy genes, the reduction in cellular energy production should be directly proportional to the number of mutant mtDNA molecules in the cell.

Given the phenomenon of the high rate of mutation of mtDNA, heteroplasmy, and replicative segregation, one would predict that women could give rise to lines of descendants differing in the severity of their disease. One line would become less severely affected from generation to generation, as the normal mitochondria becomes predominant, whereas the other would worsen as the mutation became prevalent. Thus, heteroplasmy provides the mechanism by which not all offspring of a carrier female will receive the mutation.

The clinical profile of LHON has been well established since first described in 1871 by Leber [32]. Rapid loss of central vision occurs primarily in male patients during early adult life. Age of onset of visual dysfunction is usually between 18 and 30 years, with involvement of one eye and then the second within several days or a few weeks. There is a male predominance, ranging from 60 to 90%. Color vision is affected early and visual fields demonstrate central or centrocecal defects.

In 1973, Smith and associates [33] reported the classic ophthalmoscopic findings in acute LHON: (1) circumpapillary telangiectatic microangiography; (2) swelling of the nerve fiber layer around the disc (pseudoedema); and (3) absence of leakage from the disc or peripapillary region on fluorescein angiography. This ophthalmoscopic picture may not always be seen by clinicians, and only optic atrophy with nerve fiber layer loss may remain. Recently, Lopez and Smith [34] reported that the neurovascular abnormalities may not be present in acute LHON. The diagnosis of Leber's disease can be made by finding typical circumpapillary telangiectatic microangiopathy in symptomatic or asymptomatic family members. The authors concluded that "the pathology of this disease is not in the ophthalmoscopically visible microvasculature." This conclusion is also supported by the fact that the fundus changes may be visible long before vision is lost and are found in unaffected family members [35]. The microangiopathic telangiectasias are an associated genetic marker for LHON [36].

It has long been recognized that the inheritance of LHON does not follow Mendelian principles [37–39]. Genealogical studies of carrier rates and expectancy of involvement of women are much higher than those predicted for a sex-linked recessive disease [40, 41]. A variety of other theories have been proposed, including transplacental infection, the role of slow viruses, and possible defects of cyanide metabolism.

In 1988, Wallace and associates [42] identified a mitochondrial mutation causing LHON in 9 of 11 independent pedigrees. A single nucleotide change at position 11778 in mtDNA converts codon 340 of NADH dehydrogenase subunit 4 from an arginine to a histidine. NADH dehydrogenase is the first enzyme in the electron transfer pathway and leads to a reduced complex I function in oxidative phosphorylation (see Fig 1). This mtDNA mutation has been confirmed by other investigators [43, 44].

The 11778 mutation eliminates a restriction endonuclease site in a patient's mtDNA. One molecular biological technique, termed *restriction enzymatic analysis,* can detect the mutation, but care must be taken to avoid a false-positive result. Because mtDNA mutates at 5 to 10 times the rate of nucleic DNA, there is an increased chance of a false-positive result from a harmless polymorphism [31].

Initially, most investigators found LHON mutations to be homoplasmic, but recently patients with the 11778 mutation have been found to be heteroplasmic. Holt and colleagues [45] reported one such group of patients, with varying proportions of normal and mutant mtDNA. These investigators found that the relative proportion of mutant and normal mtDNA correlated with risk of developing clinical LHON. Lott and co-workers [46] were able to demonstrate in one family that the proportion of mtDNA progressively increased from grandmother to mother to blind son. In addition, many sporadic cases of LHON occur in patients who have heteroplasmic unaffected maternal relatives. These facts suggest some cases of LHON may be a result of a mutation that has become sufficiently enriched by replicative segregation to result in clinical disease.

Much remains unexplained, however, about mutation 11778 and the etiology of LHON. Only a proportion of LHON families have this mutation. Morris [30] estimated from published cases and his own patients that only 29 of 47 families (62%) have the mutation. Further, it remains difficult to explain why all individuals with predominantly mutant mtDNA as measured in the blood do not lose vision. Possibly, although they have predominantly abnormal mtDNA in their blood, they may have predominantly normal mtDNA in their optic nerves. Another difficult question is why patients born with LHON are born homoplasmic for the mutation yet do not lose vision until later in life. One explanation for the delayed expression of the mutation is that although energy production in the optic nerve is reduced, it is not eliminated. As long as energy production is sufficient for cellular needs, the nerve will continue to function. The damage from reduced energy production may be cumulative during life with visual loss only occurring when sufficient nerve fibers die. The preponderance of LHON occurring in men still remains unexplained. Morris [30] believes there may be a different tolerance to complex I deficiency in the male and female optic nerve, although Chen and co-workers [47] failed to demonstrate the presence of a modifying X-linked gene.

What are the practical implications of the discovery of the mtDNA mutation in LHON? One obvious answer is an aid in the diagnosis of this optic neuropathy. The test is not infallible, however; only approximately 60% of familial cases involve this mutation, yet a positive result has obvious value. Detection of this mutation in asymptomatic individuals will also aid in genetic counseling. Some believe dietary advice may be helpful and provide a list of contraindicated food stuffs containing materials that may affect the process of oxidative phosphorylation. One example would be cyanide, and patients should be advised to stop smoking tobacco.

In many respects, the mtDNA mutation discovered by Wallace and co-workers [42] raises as many questions as answers regarding the etiology of LHON. Yet, this is hopefully the first step in identification of the defects causing this condition, and may lead to metabolic or genetic therapies resulting in a genuine cure.

■ Traumatic Optic Neuropathy: Diagnosis and Management

Nicholas J. Volpe, M.D., Simmons Lessell, M.D., and Lanning B. Kline, M.D.

The association between blunt forehead trauma and optic nerve blindness has been well recognized for many years; Hippocrates noted that "dimness of vision occurs in injuries to the brow and those placed slightly above" [48]. Despite this well-recognized association, considerable controversy exists in the modern medical literature concerning the appropriate diagnosis and management of visual loss occurring after closed head trauma.

Indirect optic nerve trauma is a clinical diagnosis and is defined by Walsh and Hoyt [49] as "traumatic loss of vision which occurs without external or initial ophthalmoscopic evidence of injury to the eye or its nerve." Although simply and explicitly defined, the accurate clinical diagnosis of indirect optic nerve trauma is often a formidable challenge. Ophthalmologists are often confronted with patients with multisystem injuries and an altered level of consciousness. Information concerning past ocular history and onset of blindness may be impossible to obtain. Although pupillary findings and ophthalmoscopic information are easily obtained, important information (e.g., visual acuity, color vision, visual fields) essential to the diagnosis of optic neuropathy is often unavailable. After making the diagnosis the treatment team is confronted with three disparate methods of treatment, all reported in the literature to have proven benefit in certain cases. Physicians must promptly decide on either expectant observation, treatment with steroids, or optic canal decompression. Certain guidelines are generally agreed on, but the decision is largely made on the basis of individual or institutional bias. Central to this controversy is a poor understanding of the pathogenesis of what is likely a disease of multifactorial origin with an unpredictable course. Because the disease occurs infrequently and treatment approaches are variable, there has never been a well-designed, randomized, and prospective clinical study. Physicians are often confronted with these injuries in young patients and families will often demand therapy regardless of their understanding of the potential risks and benefits.

Historical Perspective

Indirect optic nerve trauma was poorly understood until the late nineteenth century. At that time the loss of vision with blunt forehead trauma was localized to the optic nerve. In the early twentieth century, Cohen [50] and Pringle [51] were the first to question the pathogenesis and recognized that bony fracture was not required for indirect nerve trauma. In fact, in Pringle's large autopsy study there were no patients identified with bony fragments impinging on the nerve [51]. Traquair and associates [52] noticed a higher incidence of altitudinal defects in patients with indirect nerve injury and postulated a vascular etiology. Hughes [53] examined two cases histopathologically and found that although the nerves appeared grossly normal, there was necrosis in a triangle-shaped distribution and concluded that vascular insufficiency resulted from stretching on the nerve. He also recognized that visual loss can occur without fracture [53]. In 1963 Seitz [54] reported histopathological study of a case in which no vascular insult was noted but where nerve death occurred at the point where the nerve entered the cranial cavity. This finding supported the notion that shearing forces at the time of the impact may be an important factor. Finally, Walsh and Lindenberg [55] examined 140 nerves of patients with head trauma and concluded that the optic nerve could be damaged in several ways. Immediate posttrauma events could include: hemorrhage into the optic nerve, frank tears in the intraosseous portion of the nerve, and contusion necrosis. They believed these events resulted in changes that were irreversible. They described a second series of changes that could occur in the period following the trauma, and these include: edema, necrosis secondary to vascular disturbance or compromise, and necrosis from vascular occlusion. They concluded that the most important etiological factors were primary contusion necrosis and, secondarily, localized necrosis from damage to small nutrient vessels. As will be seen in the discussion that follows, these theories, reported 30 years ago, are still the basic framework to our understanding of indirect optic nerve trauma and its treatment.

Anatomical Considerations

The intracanalicular portion of the optic nerve is the segment most apt to be damaged by indirect trauma. This portion of the optic nerve is 10 mm long and measures 4 mm in cross-section. The optic canal lies between the two bases of the lesser sphenoid wing. From the orbit the canal extends posteriorly and medially and averages 9.22 mm in length (range, 5.5–11.5 mm) [56]. Contents of the optic canal include the optic nerve, meninges, the ophthalmic artery, and the postganglionic sympathetic fibers. Within the canal the optic nerve is immobilized by its dura, which is fixed to the surrounding periosteum and bone. Blood supply to the optic nerve is from penetrating pial branches of the ophthalmic and carotid arteries. The medial wall of the optic canal is on average 0.21 mm thick [56], and the distal portion of the canal (closest to the orbit) is the narrowest in cross-section and has the thickest bony walls. Four percent of normal patients have no bone medially and the nerve is separated from the sphenoid sinus only by sinus mucosa and dura [56].

Mechanism and Pathophysiology of Indirect Optic Nerve Injury

Indirect optic nerve injuries can be divided into two categories: anterior, in which funduscopic abnormalities are evident; and posterior, wherein the fundus initially appears normal. In anterior nerve injury the intraocular optic nerve (optic disc) or that portion of the intraorbital segment containing the central retinal artery is involved. In all instances, ophthalmoscopic abnormalities are visible. There may be a central retinal artery occlusion with an edematous retina, a pale disc, thread-like arterioles, visible sludging of blood flow in the retinal vasculature, and a cherry red spot in the macula. In other instances, retinal vascular spasm without thrombosis, and venous obstructive retinopathy have been observed [53]. Traumatic ischemic optic neuropathy with a diffusely swollen disc and the remainder of the fundus normal in appearance has also been reported [57, 58]. Varying degrees of avulsion of the intraocular nerve from the globe may also be seen after head trauma. Anterior marginal tears are characterized by optic nerve dysfunction with a hemorrhage at the disc margin, which rarely exceeds more than one-third of its circumference [53]. Within two weeks the hemorrhage resolves, leaving a heavily pigmented scar at the disc margin, and, subsequently, disc pallor (often mild) is evident. In general there is good correlation between the visual field defect and the visible abnormality at the disc margin. Visual acuity is variable but is usually poor. Infrequently, complete avulsion of the optic nerve may occur leading to total blindness [59].

The diagnosis of posterior optic nerve damage is made when there is evidence of optic nerve dysfunction without funduscopic abnormalities and without evidence of chiasmal injury. Optic disc pallor develops four to eight weeks after head trauma. Posterior indirect optic nerve injury can occur when the head moving forward is suddenly decelerated and the momentum of the eyeball is still forward. Sudden deceleration occurs when one of the facial eminences strikes a fixed object. The intraorbital portion of the optic nerve is spared from injury in this setting because of its relative laxity in the orbit and the protection offered by the surrounding fat. Although somewhat limited by the attachments of the extraocular muscles to the annulus of Zinn, the movement of the eyeball still places shearing and tearing forces on the fixed intracanalicular portion of the nerve. The intracranial optic nerve is less likely to be involved because of the limitation of shearing forces by the fixed intracanalicular nerve and because it is well protected by the surrounding brain and bone.

Anderson and colleagues [60] performed interferometric holographic analyses of human skulls after forces were applied to the malar eminences of cadaveric human skulls. The technique is used to analyze surface disturbances (without fractures) in bones with respect to surface loading. They demonstrated that forces applied to the frontal and malar eminences are transmitted to the area of the optic foramen. These forces alone without fracture were believed to be sufficient to cause compression, contusion, or stretching of the intracanalicular nerve. This finding may help to explain why indirect optic nerve trauma is more common with blows to the brow and cheek rather than to other parts of the head. The injury is not thought to occur in a contrecoup fashion. Turner [61] recognized that indirect nerve trauma did not typically occur in blows and decelerative injuries involving other parts of the head. In summary, damaging forces can arise from both eyeball momentum and transmitted bony surface disturbances.

The sequence of events that occurs subsequent to the force on the nerve is less clear, but vascular insufficiency is common to many theories. A normal ophthalmoscopic examination in acute traumatic optic neuropathy rules out retinal ischemia and overt damage to the central retinal artery. Shearing forces may cause frank rupture, thrombosis or spasm of small arterioles, hemorrhage, and infarction. Subsequently, edema of the nerve and compression within the optic canal develops. This compression will further compromise nutrient vessels. Alternatively, shearing forces on the nerve may cause edema, which in turn causes elevated intracanalicular pressure, compression, and ischemia without an intermediary vascular event. Ramsey [62] examined one such case in which a postmortem examination of the optic nerve was done four days after injury and revealed a totally infarcted nerve without evidence of vascular compromise. Edmund and Godtfredsen [63] examined 22 cases histopathologically and concluded that damage to small nutrient vessels is important in disease pathogenesis.

Although the microscopic events outlined probably occur in some form in almost all cases, certain optic nerve injuries are caused by "macroscopic" events. Shearing forces may cause extensive hemorrhage into the optic nerve sheath, tearing or irreversible stress of nerve fibers, or contusion necrosis.

Anterior indirect optic nerve injury can result in optic disc swelling and a retinal appearance suggestive of a central retinal vein occlusion [64]. In these reported cases, neuroimaging studies demonstrated an enlarged optic nerve with blood in the subarachnoid space surrounding the nerve [64, 65]. Release of this blood surgically through an opening in the dura was associated with a dramatic improvement in vision.

Hemorrhage may also have a role in certain cases of posterior indirect optic nerve injury. Hemorrhage may be within the nerve or within the sheath. Hemorrhage within the sheath may be intradural, subdural, or subarachnoid. The result is a hematoma causing optic nerve compression. Niho and co-workers [66] reported decompression of intradural hemorrhage in two patients, resulting in minimal improvement of visual function in both. Hammer and Ambos [67] reported four cases in which a transfrontal approach was used and a "hematoma of the optic nerve sheath" was found in each case. All patients reportedly achieved complete recovery of vision after evacuation of the hematoma.

There is no doubt that a small number of patients have compromise from direct compression by a fractured bony fragment. In certain cases, the resulting tears of the nerve or immediate contusion necrosis are unlikely to be amenable to treatment. One would think that compression by a bony fragment is perhaps the "most treatable" form of indirect optic nerve trauma; however, only a small number of such cases are documented in the literature [62,

68–71]. Fractures may involve the optic canal, the anterior clinoid process, and the orbital roof. In one case reported by Hooper [69], the intracranial portion of the optic nerve was contused by a fractured and displaced anterior clinoid process, and there was no improvement in vision after decompression. Kennerdell and colleagues [68] and Schmaltz and Schurmann [72] documented cases of visual improvement after surgical removal of a compressive bony fragment. Although there are some cases of bony compression or hemorrhage, a significant number of cases fall into the category in which microscopic events subsequent to the injury induce optic neuropathy. It is the unpredictable course of these patients that clinicians hope to alter.

Clinical Features of Indirect Traumatic Optic Neuropathy

As with other eye injuries, indirect optic nerve trauma most frequently affects men in the second and third decade. In 1938, Davidson [73] reported that falls were the most common setting for indirect nerve trauma. Noble and McFadzean [74] reported that 88% of their cases were caused by falls onto the head and motor vehicle accidents. Regardless of the exact setting of the accident, approximately 90% of patients in whom indirect optic nerve trauma develops experience blunt trauma to the brow or malar eminence with evidence of soft tissue contusion on examination [53, 74]. The essential findings on examination included loss of vision and a sluggish pupil demonstrating a relative afferent defect on swinging flashlight testing. Often there is associated epistaxis and concussion. Lessell [75] found that 27 of 33 patients had loss of consciousness (eight were unresponsive for more than 24 hours) and that this was not an important prognostic factor for visual recovery.

During evaluation of these patients, careful eye examination should be carried out by an ophthalmologist. In alert and verbal patients, Snellen or Rosenbaum near acuity should be recorded. No light perception should be confirmed with indirect ophthalmoscopy. Pupillary responses are of critical importance and should be carefully tested, and, if possible, afferent pupillary defects should be graded with neutral density filters. After reviewing 22 cases of optic nerve injury after head trauma, Edmund and Godtfredsen [63] concluded that pupillary response to light is the most reliable sign of the extent of optic nerve injury. Visual field defects will fall into the categories of central scotoma and nerve fiber bundle defects and are essential to rule out homonymous and bitemporal hemianopias. Direct and indirect ophthalmoscopy should be performed to rule out local eye trauma and direct optic nerve injury. Acutely, the optic nerve should appear normal.

Visual evoked response (VER) may be used adjunctively to document nerve conduction delays, especially in unresponsive patients. Feinsod and Auerbach [76], using a combination of the electroretinogram and VER, examined 75 patients with acute head injury. Of these, 38 suffered optic nerve injury. They found that there was usually good correlation between the initial VER and the ultimate visual acuity. In comatose patients, VER can be used to assess optic nerve function accurately; unfortunately, its availability is limited and it is not often practically performed in the setting of acute head trauma.

The presence or absence of facial and optic canal fractures should be confirmed by high-resolution CT with 1.5 mm sections in both the coronal and axial planes. The incidence of canal fractures is highly variable in the existing clinical series. Kline and associates [77], in their 1984 review, found a range of 1 to 30% of optic canal fractures in American and European studies. Since that time, series reported by Lessell [75] and Noble and McFadzean [74] found optic canal fractures in 21 and 20% of cases, respectively. In contrast, the report from Japan by Fukado [78] documented optic canal fractures in 460 of 500 patients (92%). It is difficult to explain the high incidence of fractures in Fukado's cases, as well as the lack of bilateral cases, the uniform improvement in all his patients treated with decompression, and, finally, the sheer number of cases he treated.

The presence or absence of fractures on CT will not dictate therapy except in instances of obvious bony fragment compression of the nerve. CT may also demonstrate other abnormalities, including orbital lesions, foreign bodies, and subperiosteal fluid collections. Shaked and colleagues [79] reported a case in which CT demonstrated right proptosis and stretching of the optic nerve due to orbital edema. Anderson and co-workers [60] reported a case in which CT revealed a mass in the superonasal orbit that proved to be a subperiosteal hematoma.

Although recognized as inferior for evaluating bone, MRI is valuable when evaluating the intracanalicular and intracranial optic nerve. With increasing availability and clinical use, MRI is likely to be recognized as an important adjunct to CT in evaluating indirect optic nerve trauma.

Cases of anterior optic nerve injury should undergo orbital ultrasound as well. Hupp and co-workers [64] and Guy and associates [65] reported cases in which progressive visual loss after head trauma was associated with venous obstructive retinopathy and progressive enlargement of the optic nerve sheath on B-scan ultrasonography and CT. In these cases there was improvement in vision following sheath fenestration of the intraorbital optic nerve.

Treatment of Indirect Optic Nerve Trauma

After obtaining all of the clinical and radiographical information it is still impossible to predict which patients will spontaneously improve, which patients will progressively lose vision, and which will not recover at all. It should be emphasized that all reports of treatment methods are difficult to evaluate because they are uncontrolled and nonrandomized. Table 3 summarizes the results in series in which nonsurgical therapy was used. Eleven of Davidson's 37 patients enjoyed spontaneous improvement [73]. Hughes [53] found that six of the 36 patients who initially had no light perception improved spontaneously. Lessell [75] had two of five patients with no light perception improve and gain useful vision without intervention. Recently, Wolin and Lavin [80] reported four patients with no light perception from indirect optic nerve trauma who recovered vision (three were better than 20/50) without or before steroid therapy was instituted. It should be noted that three of the four patients had associated eye injuries, although none were judged to be serious enough to cause no light perception. It is therefore well established that some patients will improve without intervention. The possibility does exist that they would have improved more or faster with therapy. On the other hand, there are

Table 3 *Nonsurgical Therapy of Indirect Optic Nerve Injury*

Authors, Year, Ref	No. Patients	No. Improved	No. Not Improved	Comment
Davidson, 1938, [73]	37	11	26	. . .
Turner, 1943, [61]	46	23	23	. . .
Hooper, 1951, [69]	17	5	12	. . .
Anderson et al, 1982, [60]	2	2	0	"Megadose" steroids
Tang et al, 1986, [88]	13	5	8	No treatment
	5	1	4	"Therapeutic dose of steroids"
	11	4	7	"Megadose" steroids
Millesi et al, 1988, [89]	7	4	3	No specific treatment
	2	1	1	Intravenous steroids
Lessell, 1989, [75]	25	5	20	No specific treatment
	4	1	3	Steroids; dosage not given
Wolin and Lavin, 1990, [80]	4	4	0	"Megadose" steroids in 3 patients
Seiff, 1990, [90]	15	5	10	No specific treatment
	21	13	8	"Megadose" steroids
Spoor et al, 1990, [81]	22	19	3	"Megadose" steroids

patients in whom both steroids and decompressive surgery were used without benefit [75, 81].

Rationale for Treatment Matsuzaki and colleagues [82] measured VERs in monkeys that had either a shearing injury to the nerve or ligation of the nerve for up to 10 days. They found that although temporarily extinguished, recovery could always be demonstrated despite the presence of degenerative changes on histopathological examination. What can be done to minimize tissue damage? Edema is the well-recognized response of the central nervous system to trauma, and, as discussed previously, likely has an important role in traumatic optic neuropathy. Steroids have an important part in the management of central nervous system edema resulting from tumors and infection, but their role in the setting of trauma is less clear. In an animal study, Harrison and associates [83] demonstrated the usefulness of megadoses of steroids in reducing brain edema after carotid ligation. Bracken and co-workers [84], in a randomized, prospective, double-blind study, evaluated the use of megadose methylprednisolone within eight hours of acute spinal cord injury. They found that megadose steroids significantly reduced the incidence of paralysis and other disabilities. In an earlier report [85] they were unable to demonstrate a significant effect from lower steroid doses.

The mechanism of action of megadose steroids is not entirely known. It is possible that steroids reduce microcirculatory spasm, edema, and nerve cell death. They may reduce both intraneural and extraneural edema, thereby reducing swelling, improving blood flow, and reducing cell damage from ischemia. Spoor and colleagues [81], based on the work of Braughler and Hall [86], recommend steroid doses for treatment of indirect optic nerve trauma of either dexamethasone (6 mg/kg body weight) or methylprednisolone (30 mg/kg body weight) as an initial bolus followed two hours later and then every six hours by half of the initial bolus. Similar doses are recommended by Anderson and co-workers [60]. The major disadvantages of steroid therapy are its many well-known side effects and the theoretical possibility that their use could delay other therapy (i.e., nerve decompression).

The rationale for surgical treatment is simple. Visual loss from compressive optic neuropathy is reversible. To the extent that edema and swelling elevate pressure within the optic canal and on the nerve, there is a compressive component. It is this compression that surgeons try to relieve. In other situations where a compressive hematoma or bony fragment is identified, evacuation or removal is required to relieve compression. The goal of decompression is to remove approximately half the circumference of the bony canal for the entire length of the canal. The need for incision of the nerve sheath is debated without consensus among surgeons performing this technique. Decompression can be accomplished in many ways, including transcranial, transorbital, transethmoidal, transantral-transethmoidal, and endonasal-transethmoidal. Transethmoidal surgery was first described by Sewall in 1926 [87]. Descriptions of each technique are beyond the scope of this discussion, but suffice it to say that all require microsurgical technique, and the techniques that do not require craniotomy are associated with less morbidity and mortality. The anatomy, especially the proximity of the optic nerve to the bony canal, carotid artery, and cavernous sinus, mandates that surgeons use extreme care and perform prior cadaver dissections before clinical application. Complications of surgery are rare but include damage to the optic nerve, cerebrospinal fluid rhinorrhea, and meningitis.

There are several studies that support the use of surgical decompression. Reported series of surgical decompression are summarized in Table 4. The greatest support for optic nerve decompression comes from the Japanese literature. Series reported by Fukado [78], Fujitani and colleagues [97], and Niho and associates [93] demonstrate a high success rate with nerve decompression and recommend it almost routinely. All of Fukado's 400 patients improved with decompression [78]. Fujitani and colleagues [97] limit surgical indications to all patients with initial no light perception vision and those that do not improve to 20/40 within three weeks on oral prednisone. They found that none of the nine blind eyes improved on conservative therapy, but seven of the 28 blind eyes undergoing decompressive surgery improved. Niho and associates [93] reported that 20 of 25 patients improved with decompression.

Additional support for surgical decompression comes from isolated cases in the literature of patients who worsened or failed to improve on steroids, who were then successfully managed by decompression. Case reports by Kennerdell and co-workers [68], Spoor and Mathog [100], and Spoor and colleagues [81] document that incomplete or temporary improvement on steroids

Table 4 *Surgical Therapy of Indirect Optic Nerve Injury*

Authors, Year, Ref	No. Patients	Time Between Injury and Operation	No. Improved	No. Not Improved
Pringle, 1922, [91]	3	2–4 weeks	0	3
Daum, 1951, [92]	12	1–72 days	0	12
Hooper, 1951, [69]	4	18 hr–18 mo	1	3
Niho et al, 1961, [66]	7	5–263 days	5	2
Hughes, 1962, [53]	5	20 hr–2 mo	0	5
Edmund and Godtfredsen, 1963, [63]	6	. . .	1	5
Imachi et al, 1969, [70]	61	. . .	45	16
Niho et al, 1970, [93]	25	. . .	20	5
Schmaltz and Schurmann, 1971, [72]	13	. . .	1	12
Hammer and Ambos, 1971, [67]	4	"Within one week"	4	0
Fukado, 1975, [78]	400	Less than 7 to greater than 90 days[a]	400	0
Goldware et al, 1980, [94]	2	36 hr–10 weeks	2	0
Karnick et al, 1981, [95]	10	Less than 1 week to more than 1 month[a]	2	8
Brihaye, 1981, [96]	56	. . .	7	49
Anderson et al, 1982, [60][a]	4	12–48 hr	1	3
Tang et al, 1986, [88]	8	. . .	2	6
Fujitani et al, 1989, [97]	28	. . .	7	21
Waga et al, 1988, [98]	22	"Within 21 days"	11	11
Millesi et al, 1988, [89]	3	12–24 hr	0	3
Lessell, 1989, [75][a]	4	36–72 hr	3	1
Joseph et al, 1990, [99][a]	14	1–5 days	11	3

[a]Corticosteroids used as well.

was followed by further clinical improvement after decompression. Lessell [75] reported clinical improvement in three of four patients treated with decompression and conventional non-"megadose" steroids. In another series, three patients who failed to improve on megadose steroids also failed to improve with decompression [60]. In the only western series in which extracranial optic nerve decompression was applied to all noncomatose patients seen at one center with optic nerve trauma, Joseph and associates [99] reported that 11 of 14 patients improved. This series included five patients who were blind initially; three of these patients improved, with two reaching better than 20/50 final acuity. There was no morbidity or mortality. This study has been criticized because of the simultaneous use of nonstandardized doses of systemic steroids and the exclusion of comatose patients [101, 102].

More conservative, less invasive treatment methods are more easily applied. Megadose steroid therapy is relatively noninvasive and can be administered immediately. In a series of 22 eyes treated with megadose steroids, Spoor and colleagues [81] reported clinical improvement in 19. Seiff [90] looked at a retrospective series of 36 patients and found that 13 of 21 treated with high-dose intravenous dexamethasone (1 mg/kg/day; note that these doses are less than the megadoses outlined previously) improved. They noted that steroid-treated patients seemed to improve faster and more completely. Anderson and co-workers [60] reported clinical improvement in three of six patients treated with megadose steroids. They concluded that decompression should be reserved for delayed visual loss after frontal head trauma that is unresponsive to megadose steroid therapy and in cases in which initial return of vision with megadose steroids is followed by visual decrease while still on steroids.

■ Conclusions

Indirect optic nerve trauma resulting from closed head injury is a relatively rare condition of uncertain pathogenesis. Many patients will enjoy spontaneous recovery, whereas others remain blind despite the heroic efforts of their physicians. A significant number of patients have a reversible and sometimes progressive course that, although unpredictable, can be altered. To date, there is no general consensus concerning treatment, and managing physicians make individual decisions based on their clinical experience. We use the following guidelines in designing treatment strategies [103].

1. If indirect optic nerve trauma is diagnosed in the setting of blunt head trauma and there are no medical contraindications, megadose steroids should be given as soon as possible.
2. Once on steroids, if there is continued deterioration, or improvement and then deterioration, optic nerve decompression should be performed.
3. Once on steroids, if there is no improvement after 12 to 24 hours, decompression may be indicated but must be individualized by the treating physicians.
4. If the patient relapses on discontinuation of systemic steroids, surgical decompression should be considered.
5. Decompression should not be used as an elective procedure in unconscious patients who are unable to cooperate with examination and unable to understand preoperatively the risks and benefits of surgery.
6. Decompression may be used primarily in a comatose patient with indirect optic nerve trauma who is undergoing other craniofacial surgery.
7. If an obvious compressive lesion (such as hematoma or bone fragment) is present, surgical decompression should be performed.
8. Recovery from no light perception can occur, and because it is difficult to determine if this loss occurred at the moment of impact, patients with no light perception should be treated as others.
9. Transethmoidal surgery is as effective as transcranial surgery and is probably associated with less morbidity.

These approaches should only be guidelines and are not based on personal clinical data but on the information available in the literature. The real answer to treatment questions will come from a randomized, prospective, multicenter study with a control group or, more feasibly, from a central data bank of treated cases. As suggested by Kline and associates [77], each institution must identify a team of physicians to treat patients in a uniform way. The team should include a neuro-ophthalmologist, an otolaryngologist, a neurosurgeon, and a radiologist, and should have a previously defined protocol to which they adhere closely. With time and more uniform application of the available alternatives, the best treatment will hopefully be identified.

■ References

1. Sergott RC, Grossman RI, Savino PJ, et al. The syndrome of paradoxical worsening of dural-cavernous sinus arteriovenous malformations. Ophthalmology 1987;94:205–212
2. Winward KE, Hamed LM, Glaser JS. The spectrum of optic nerve disease in human immunodeficiency virus infections. Am J Ophthalmol 1989;107:373–380
3. Mansour AM. Neuro-ophthalmic findings in acquired immunodeficiency syndrome. J Clin Neuro-ophthalmol 1990;10:167–174
4. Kardon RH, Denison CE, Brown CK, Thompson HS. Critical evaluation of the cocaine test in the diagnosis of Horner's syndrome. Arch Ophthalmol 1990;108: 384–387
5. Cremer SA, Thompson HS, Digre KB, Kardon RH. Hydroxyamphetamine mydriasis in Horner's syndrome. Am J Ophthalmol 1990;110:71–76
6. Fisher CM, Ojemann RG, Roberson GH. Spontaneous dissection of cervicocerebral arteries. Can J Neurol 1978;5:9–19
7. Mokri B, Sundt TM, Houser OW, Piepgras DG. Spontaneous dissection of the cervical internal carotid artery. Ann Neurol 1986;19:126–138
8. Bogousslavsky J, Despland PA, Regli F. Spontaneous carotid dissection with acute stroke. Arch Neurol 1987;44:137–140
9. Kline LB, Vitek JJ, Ramon BC. Painful Horner's syndrome due to spontaneous carotid artery dissection. Ophthalmology 1987;94:226–230
10. Newman NJ, Kline LB, Leifer D, Lessell S. Ocular stroke and carotid artery dissection. Neurology 1989;39:1462–1464
11. Maitland CG, Black JL, Smith WA. Abducens nerve palsy due to spontaneous dissection of the internal carotid artery. Arch Neurol 1983;40:448–449
12. Anderson RMcD, Schechter MM. A case of spontaneous dissecting aneurysm of the internal carotid artery. J Neurol Neurosurg Psychiatry 1959;22:195–201
13. Brice JG, Crampton MR. Spontaneous dissecting aneurysm of the cervical internal carotid artery. Br Med J 1964;2:790–792
14. Goldberg HI, Grissman RI, Gomori JM, et al. Cervical internal carotid artery dissecting hemorrhage: diagnosis using MR. Radiology 1986;158:157–161
15. Anderson DR, Trobe JD, Hood TW, Gebarski SS. Optic tract injury after anterior temporal lobectomy. Ophthalmology 1989;96:1065–1070
16. Trobe JD. Third nerve palsy and the pupil. Footnotes to the rule. Arch Ophthalmol 1988;106:601–602
17. Lorentzen SE. Drusen of the optic disk. Acta Ophthalmol 1966;90(suppl):9–180
18. Savino PJ, Glaser JS, Rosenberg MA. A clinical analysis of pseudopapilledema. II. Visual fields. Arch Ophthalmol 1979;97:71–75

19. Beck RW, Corbett JJ, Thompson HS, Sergott RC. Decreased visual acuity from optic disc drusen. Arch Ophthalmol 1985;103:1155–1159
20. Smith TS, Baker RS. Perimetric findings in functional disorders using automated techniques. Ophthalmology 1987;94:1562–1566
21. Cogan DC. Alzheimer syndromes. Am J Ophthalmol 1987;104:183–184
22. Sadun AA, Borchert M, Devita E, et al. Assessment of visual impairment in patients with Alzheimer's disease. Am J Ophthalmol 1987;104:113–120
23. Katz B, Rimmer S. Ophthalmologic manifestations of Alzheimer's disease. Surv Ophthalmol 1989;34:31–43
24. Lee WH, Bookstein R, Heng F, et al. Human retinoblastoma susceptibility gene. Cloning, identification, and sequence. Science 1987;235:1394–1399
25. Wright AF, Bhattacharga SS, Craig IW, et al. Recombinant DNA mapping of retinitis pigmentosa genes. In: Piatigorsky J, Shinohara T, Zelenka PS, eds. Molecular biology of the eye. Genes, vision and ocular disease. New York: Alan J Liss, 1988:293–304
26. Nathans J, Piantanider TP, Eddy RL, et al. Molecular genetics of inherited variation in human color vision. Science 1986;232:203–210
27. Inana G, Hotta Y, Zintz C, et al. Molecular genetics of gyrate atrophy. In: Piatigorsky J, Shinohara T, Zelenka PS, eds. Molecular biology of the eye. Genes, vision and ocular disease. New York: Alan J Liss, 1988:317–328
28. Mitchell GA, Brody LC, Sipila I, et al. At least two mutant alleles of ornithine aminotransferase cause gyrate atrophy of the choroid and retina. Proc Natl Acad Sci USA 1989;86:197
29. Newman NJ, Wallace DC. Mitochondria and Leber's hereditary optic neuropathy. Am J Ophthalmol 1990;109:726–730
30. Morris M. Mitochondrial mutations in neuro-ophthalmological diseases. J Clin Neuro-ophthalmol 1990;10:159–166
31. Johns DR. The molecular genetics of Leber's hereditary optic neuropathy. Arch Ophthalmol 1990;108:1405–1407
32. Leber T. Veber hereditare und congenitulangelegte sehnervenleiden. Graefes Arch Ophthalmol 1971;17:249
33. Smith JL, Hoyt WF, Susac JO. Ocular fundus in Leber's optic neuropathy. Arch Ophthalmol 1973;90:349–354
34. Lopez PF, Smith JL. Leber's optic neuropathy. New observations. J Clin Neuro-ophthalmol 1986;6:144–152
35. Lessell S, Gise RL, Krohel GB. Bilateral optic neuropathy with remission in young men: variation on a theme by Leber? Arch Neurol 1983;40:2–6
36. Rogers JA. Leber's disease. Aust J Ophthalmol 1977;5:111–119
37. Carroll WM, Mastalgia FL. Leber's optic neuropathy. A clinical and visual evoked potential study of affected and asymptomatic members of a six generation family. Brain 1979;102:559–580
38. Seedorff T. The inheritance of Leber's disease. A genealogical follow-up study. Acta Ophthalmol 1985;63:135–145
39. Nikoskelainen E. New aspects of the genetic, etiologic and clinical puzzle of Leber's disease. Neurology 1984;34:1482–1484
40. Miller NR. The hereditary optic neuropathies. Monosymptomatic hereditary optic neuropathies. Leber's optic neuropathy. In: Miller NR. Walsh and Hoyt's clinical neuro-ophthalmology, ed. 4, vol 1. Baltimore: William & Wilkins, 1982:311–317
41. Nikoskelainen E, Savontanus ML, Wanne OP, et al. Leber's hereditary optic neuroretinopathy, a maternally inherited disease. A genealogic study in four pedigrees. Arch Ophthalmol 1987;105:665–671
42. Wallace DC, Singh G, Lott MT, et al. Mitochondrial DNA mutation associated with Leber's hereditary optic neuropathy. Science 1988;242:1427–1430

43. Yoneda M, Tsuji S, Yamauchi T, et al. Mitochondrial DNA mutation in family with Leber's hereditary optic neuropathy. Lancet 1989;1:1076–1077
44. Parker WD, Oleg CA, Parks JK. A defect in mitochondrial electron-transport activity (NADH-coenzyme Q oxidoreductase) in Leber's hereditary optic neuropathy. N Engl J Med 1989;320:1331–1333
45. Holt IJ, Miller DH, Harding AE. Genetic heterogeneity and mitochondrial DNA heteroplasmy in Leber's hereditary optic neuropathy. J Med Genet 1989;26: 739–743
46. Lott MT, Voljavec S, Wallace DC. Variable genotype of Leber's hereditary optic neuropathy patients. Am J Ophthalmol 1990;109:625–631
47. Chen JD, Cox I, Denten MJ. Preliminary exclusion of an X-linked gene in Leber's optic atrophy by linkage analysis. Hum Genet 1989;82:203–207
48. Chadwick J, Munn WN. The medical works of Hippocrates. Oxford, England: Blackwell, 1950
49. Walsh FB, Hoyt WF. Clinical neuro-ophthalmology. Baltimore: Williams & Wilkins, 1969:2375–2380
50. Cohen M. The value of eye manifestations complicating fractured skull. Arch Ophthalmol 1917;46:705–716
51. Pringle JH. Monocular blindness following diffused violence to the skull: its causation and treatment. Br J Surg 1916;4:373–385
52. Traquair HM, Dott NM, Russell WR. Traumatic lesion of the optic chiasma. Brain 1935;58:398–411
53. Hughes B. Indirect injury of the optic nerves and chiasm. Bull Johns Hopkins Hosp 1963;11:98–126
54. Seitz R. Atiologie und Genese der akuten Erblindung als Folge stumpfer Schadelverletzungen: Ein Beitrag zur Frage der exploratorischen Freilegung des Canalis opticus. Klin Monatsbl Augenheilkd 1963;143:414–429
55. Walsh FB, Lindenberg RL. Die Verandergungen des Schnerven bei indirektem Trauma. In: Entwicklung und Fortschrift in der Augenheilkunde: Forbildungskurs fur Augenaerzte Hamburg. Stuttgart, West Germany: Enke Verlag, 1963: 83–107
56. Maniscalco JE, Habal MB. Microanatomy of the optic canal. J Neurosurg 1978; 48:402–406
57. Hedges TR III, Gragoudas ES. Traumatic anterior ischemic optic neuropathy. Ann Ophthalmol 1981;13:625–628
58. Wyllie AM, Mcleod D, Cullen JF. Traumatic ischaemic optic neuropathy. Br J Ophthalmol 1972;56:851–853
59. Hillman JS, Myska V, Nissim S. Complete avulsion of the optic nerve: a clinical, angiographic, and electrodiagnostic study. Br J Ophthalmol 1975;59:503–509
60. Anderson RL, Panje WR, Gross CE. Optic nerve blindness following blunt forehead trauma. Ophthalmology 1982;89:445–455
61. Turner JWA. Indirect injury of the optic nerves. Brain 1943;66:140–151
62. Ramsey JH. Optic nerve injury in fracture of the canal. Br J Ophthalmol 1979; 63:607–610
63. Edmund J, Godtfredsen E. Unilateral optic atrophy following head injury. Acta Ophthalmol 1963;41:693–697
64. Hupp SL, Buckley EG, Byrne SF, et al. Post-traumatic venous obstructive retinopathy associated with enlarged optic nerve sheath. Arch Ophthalmol 1984;102: 254–256
65. Guy J, Sherwood M, Day AL. Surgical treatment of progressive visual loss in traumatic optic neuropathy. J Neurosurg 1989;70:799–801
66. Niho S, Yasuda K, Sato T, et al. Decompression of the optic canal by the transethmoidal route. Am J Ophthalmol 1961;51:659–665

67. Hammer VG, Ambos E. Das traumatische Optikusscheidenhamatom und seine operative Behandlunsmoglichkeit. Klin Monatsbl Augenheilkd 1971;159:818–819
68. Kennerdell JS, Amsbaugh GA, Myers EN. Transantral-ethmoidal decompression of optic canal fracture. Arch Ophthalmol 1976;94:1040–1043
69. Hooper RS. Orbital complications of head injury. Br J Surg 1951;39:126–138
70. Imachi J, Inove K, Takahashi T. Clinical and pathohistological investigations of optic nerve lesions in cases of head injuries. Jpn J Ophthalmol 1968;12:70–85
71. Obenchain TG, Killeffer FA, Stern WE. Indirect injury of the optic nerves and chiasm with closed head injury. Bull Los Angeles Neurol Soc 1973;38:13–20
72. Schmaltz B, Schurmann K. Traumatische optikuss chaden: probleme der Atiologie und der operativen Behandlung. Klin Monatsbl Augenheilkd 1971;153: 33–40
73. Davidson M. The indirect optic atrophies. Am J Ophthalmol 1938;21:7–21
74. Noble MJ, McFadzean R. Indirect injury to the optic nerves and chiasm. Neuro-ophthalmology 1987;7:341–348
75. Lessell S. Indirect optic nerve trauma. Arch Ophthalmol 1989;107:382–386
76. Feinsod M, Auerbach E. Electrophysiological examinations of the visual system in the acute phase after head injury. Eur Neurol 1973;9:56–64
77. Kline LB, Morawetz RB, Swaid SN. Indirect injury of the optic nerve. Neurosurgery 1984;14:756–764
78. Fukado Y. Results in 400 cases of surgical decompression of the optic nerve. Mod Prob Ophthalmol 1975;14:474–481
79. Shaked A, Hadani M, Feinsod M. CT and VER follow-up of reversible visual loss with fracture of the optic canal. Acta Neurochir 1982;62:91–94
80. Wolin MJ, Lavin PJM. Spontaneous visual recovery from traumatic optic neuropathy after blunt head injury. Am J Ophthalmol 1990;109:430–435
81. Spoor TC, Hartel WC, Lensink DB, Wilkinson MJ. Treatment of traumatic optic neuropathy with corticosteroids. Am J Ophthalmol 1990;110:665–669
82. Matsuzaki H, Kunita M, Kawai K. Optic nerve damage in head trauma: clinical and experimental studies. Jpn J Ophthalmol 1982;26:447–461
83. Harrison MJG, Brownbill D, Lewis PD, Ross Russel RW. Cerebral edema following carotid artery ligation in the gerbil. Arch Neurol 1973;28:389–391
84. Bracken MB, Shepard MJ, Collins WF, et al. A randomized controlled trial of methylprednisolone or naloxone in the treatment of acute spinal cord injury. N Engl J Med 1990;322:1405–1411
85. Bracken MB, Collins WF, Freeman DF, et al. Efficacy of methylprednisolone in active spinal cord injury. JAMA 1984;251:45–52
86. Braughler JM, Hall ED. Current applications of "high dose" steroid therapy for CNS injury. J Neurosurg 1985;62:806–810
87. Sewall EC. External operation in the ethmo-sphenoidal-frontal group of sinuses under local anesthesia. Technique for removal of part of the foramen wall for the relief of pressure on optic nerve. Arch Otolaryngol 1926;4:377–411
88. Tang RA, Li HK, Regner V, et al. Traumatic optic neuropathy. Analysis of 37 cases. ARVO abstracts. Supplement to Invest Ophthalmol Vis Sci. Philadelphia: JB Lippincott, 1986:102
89. Millesi W, Hollmann K, Funder J. Traumatic lesion of the optic nerve. Acta Neurochir 1988;93:50–54
90. Seiff SR. High dose corticosteroids for treatment of vision loss due to indirect injury to the optic nerve. Ophthalmic Surg 1990;21:389–395
91. Pringle JH. Atrophy of the optic nerve following diffused violence to the skull. Br Med J 1922;2:1156–1157
92. Daum S. Quoted by Walsh FB, Hoyt WF. Clinical neuro-ophthalmology. Baltimore: Williams & Wilkins, 1969:2381

93. Niho S, Niho M, Niho K. Decompression of the optic canal by the transethmoidal route and decompression of the superior orbital fissure. Can J Ophthalmol 1970;5:22–40
94. Goldware S, Sylvester R, Baker L. Delayed post-traumatic optic neuropathy with recovery after unroofing the optic canal. Neuro-ophthalmology 1980;1:77–78
95. Karnick PP, Maskati BT, Kirtane MV, Tonsekan KS. Optic nerve decompression in head injuries. J Laryngol Otol 1981;95:1135–1140
96. Brihaye J. Transcranial decompression of the optic nerve after trauma. In: Samil M, Janetta PF, ed. The cranial nerves. New York: Springer-Verlag, 1981:116–124
97. Fujitani T, Inoue K, Takahashi T, et al. Indirect traumatic optic neuropathy: visual outcome of operative and nonoperative cases. Jpn J Ophthalmol 1986; 30:125–134
98. Waga S, Kubo Y, Sakakura M. Transfrontal intradural microsurgical decompression for traumatic optic nerve injury. Acta Neurochir 1988;91:42–46
99. Joseph MP, Lessell S, Rizzo J, Momose KJ. Extracranial optic nerve decompression for traumatic optic neuropathy. Arch Ophthalmol 1990;108:1091–1093
100. Spoor TC, Mathog RH. Restoration of vision after optic canal decompression. Arch Ophthalmol 1986;104:804–806
101. Miller NR. The management of traumatic optic neuropathy. Arch Ophthalmol 1990;109:1086–1087
102. Seiff SR. Therapy for traumatic optic neuropathy. Arch Ophthalmol 1991; 109:610
103. Lessell S. Traumatic optic neuropathy and visual system injury. In: Shingleton BJ, Hersh PS, Kenyon KR, eds. Eye trauma. St Louis: Mosby Year Book, 1991: 371–379

Index

Future Issues

Volume 32, 1992

Winter (No. 1)

PEDIATRIC OPHTHALMOLOGY
Frederick A. Jakobiec, M.D., and Dimitri Azar, M.D., Guest Editors

Spring (No. 2)

RETINAL AND VITREAL SURGERY
Joseph Olk, M.D., Guest Editor

Summer (No. 3)

ORBITAL DISEASE
John Shore, M.D., Guest Editor

Fall (No. 4)

COMPLICATIONS IN OPHTHALMIC SURGERY